HEALTH CARE IN TRANSITION

STAFFING ISSUES IN MILITARY HEALTH CARE

MENTAL HEALTH PROVIDERS AND VA NURSING

HEALTH CARE IN TRANSITION

Additional books in this series can be found on Nova's website under the Series tab.

Additional e-books in this series can be found on Nova's website under the e-book tab.

HEALTH CARE IN TRANSITION

STAFFING ISSUES IN MILITARY HEALTH CARE

MENTAL HEALTH PROVIDERS AND VA NURSING

DOUGLAS PARKER
EDITOR

NOVINKA

New York

Library of Congress Cataloging-in-Publication Data

ISBN: 978-1-63482-993-9

Published by Nova Science Publishers, Inc. † New York

CONTENTS

PREFACE

Mental health providers are essential to the Department of Defense's (DOD) delivery of health care to servicemembers and other beneficiaries. DOD's need for these providers has grown as increasing numbers of servicemembers experience life-threatening combat situations. This led to congressional attention—such as the NDAA for Fiscal Year 2010, which included provisions to help DOD increase the number of mental health providers it employs. This book examines how staffing levels changed in response to congressional direction; and how DOD and the military services assess current and future needs for mental health providers. Furthermore, this book reviews the extent to which Department of Veterans Affairs medical centers (VAMC) have implemented the Veterans Health Administration's (VHA) nurse staffing methodology; and VHA oversees VAMCs' implementation and ongoing administration of the methodology.

In: Staffing Issues in Military Health Care
Editor: Douglas Parker
ISBN: 978-1-63482-993-9

Chapter 1

DEFENSE HEALTH CARE: ADDITIONAL INFORMATION NEEDED ABOUT MENTAL HEALTH PROVIDER STAFFING NEEDS*

United States Government Accountability Office

WHY GAO DID THIS STUDY

Mental health providers are essential to DOD's delivery of health care to servicemembers and other beneficiaries. DOD's need for these providers has grown as increasing numbers of servicemembers experience life-threatening combat situations. This led to congressional attention—such as the NDAA for Fiscal Year 2010, which included provisions to help DOD increase the number of mental health providers it employs.

GAO was asked to review DOD's efforts to increase its mental health provider workforce. Among other objectives, GAO examined (1) how staffing levels changed in response to congressional direction and (2) how DOD and the military services assess current and future needs for mental health providers. GAO reviewed DOD's mental health staffing estimation model and the military services' quarterly mental health provider staffing reports for

* This is an edited, reformatted and augmented version of a United States Government Accountability Office publication, No. GAO-15-184, dated January 2015.

fiscal years 2009 through 2013, the latest information available. GAO also interviewed DOD and military service officials responsible for assessing mental health staffing needs.

WHAT GAO RECOMMENDS

GAO recommends that the military services report on service-specific or supplemental processes for generating mental health provider staffing estimates and that DOD continue to refine its staffing estimation model. DOD generally concurred with these recommendations, but did not concur with two others related to the use of PHRAMS that are also included in the report. GAO continues to believe these recommendations are valid as discussed further in the report.

WHAT GAO FOUND

In response to the enactment of the National Defense Authorization Act (NDAA) for Fiscal Year 2010, the Department of Defense (DOD) military health system (MHS) increased its mental health provider staffing level by 34 percent. Specifically, DOD increased the number of mental health providers across the MHS from 4,608 providers in fiscal year 2009 to 6,186 providers in fiscal year 2013. Social workers and psychologists were the most frequently added types of mental health providers during this period.

In 2007, DOD created the Psychological Health Risk-Adjusted Model for Staffing (PHRAMS) to assess the MHS's current and future mental health provider staffing needs and DOD annually revises this model. Fiscal year 2014 marked the first time the model was used by the three military services responsible for providing health care—the Army, Air Force, and Navy—for a common purpose, which was the development of DOD's fiscal year 2016 budget request for mental health services. However, GAO found that the military services either were not using PHRAMS as the main basis of their mental health provider staffing needs estimates or were supplementing PHRAMS results with other service-specific methods. The services reported making these adjustments because PHRAMS does not account for factors that are crucial to assess mental health provider staffing needs, such as mental health providers needed for deployments. As a result, the military services' estimates of mental health provider staffing needs may not consistently reflect the beneficiary demand for mental health providers across the military services, and the current version of PHRAMS may not fully capture the military services' needs.

ABBREVIATIONS

DHA	Defense Health Agency
DOD	Department of Defense
HPSP	Health Professions Scholarship and Financial Assistance Program
MHS	military health system
MTF	military treatment facility
NCR	National Capital Region
NDAA	National Defense Authorization Act
OASD HA	Office of the Assistant Secretary of Defense for Health Affairs
PHRAMS	Psychological Health Risk-Adjusted Model for Staffing
USUHS	Uniformed Services University of the Health Sciences

* * *

January 30, 2015

The Honorable Thad Cochran
Chairman
The Honorable Richard J. Durbin
Vice Chairman
Subcommittee on Defense
Committee on Appropriations
United States Senate

Mental health providers are essential to maintaining the Department of Defense's (DOD) capability to deliver health care services.[1] As part of its mission, DOD provides a full range of medical care and services, including mental health services, at no cost to active duty military servicemembers and at either a reduced cost or no cost to other eligible beneficiaries–including dependents of servicemembers and some military retirees.[2] DOD's ability to deliver this care has been impacted by increasing numbers of servicemembers who experienced life-threatening situations in combat and their resulting need for mental health services.[3] Specifically, DOD faces significant challenges building and maintaining a mental health provider workforce–including active duty and reserve military providers and civilian and contract providers working in military medical facilities–that is capable of providing all the mental health care servicemembers and their dependents need due to nationwide shortages of mental health providers.[4] These challenges are exacerbated by the pressure to control DOD healthcare costs and the need to compete for mental health providers with other health care delivery systems throughout the nation which also face increased needs for these providers.[5]

The increased need for mental health care for servicemembers and their dependents has led to congressional attention on the recruitment and retention of qualified mental health providers to work in DOD's military health system (MHS). Specifically, the National Defense Authorization Act (NDAA) for Fiscal Year 2010 included provisions for DOD to increase its mental health capabilities by increasing the number of active duty mental health providers and to report on the appropriate number of mental health providers required to meet the mental health care needs of servicemembers, retirees, and dependents.[6]

You asked us to review DOD's efforts to increase its qualified mental health provider workforce. In this report we examine (1) the staffing levels of DOD military, civilian, and contracted mental health providers and how these staffing levels have changed in response to the NDAA for Fiscal Year 2010; (2) how DOD and the military services assess current and future needs for mental health providers; and (3) how the military services report mental health provider staffing levels and future needs to DOD.

To examine the staffing levels of DOD military, civilian, and contract mental health providers and how these staffing levels changed in response to the NDAA for Fiscal Year 2010, we analyzed quarterly mental health staffing reports for fiscal years 2009 through 2013 submitted to DOD from each military service and the National Capital Region (NCR) Medical Directorate.[7] We analyzed these reports separately and together to report current mental health provider staffing levels and compare mental health provider staffing levels from fiscal year 2009, prior to the enactment of the NDAA for Fiscal Year 2010, with such levels from fiscal year 2013. Fiscal year 2013 was the most recent fiscal year with complete data available for analysis. To ensure the reliability of these data, we interviewed Office of the Assistant Secretary of Defense for Health Affairs (OASD HA) officials responsible for collecting and analyzing these quarterly staffing reports and reviewed documentation related to the production of these reports. Based on these actions, we found information contained in these quarterly staffing reports to be sufficiently reliable for the purposes of this report.

To examine how DOD and the military services assess current and future needs for mental health providers, we interviewed officials from OASD HA, Army, Air Force, Navy, 8 the DOD Task Force on Mental Health, and the Interagency Task Force on Military and Veterans Mental Health to learn about actions taken to assess mental health provider staffing levels.[9] We also reviewed the Psychological Health Risk-Adjusted Model for Staffing (PHRAMS), DOD's mental health staffing model used to project the number and mix of health care providers needed to meet the mental health care needs of the DOD health care system—including procedure guides and year-end reports.

To examine how the military services report mental health provider staffing levels and future needs to DOD, we interviewed officials from OASD HA, Army, Air Force, Navy, and the NCR Medical Directorate to learn about their use of quarterly mental health staffing reports. We also reviewed the quarterly mental health staffing reports submitted by the military services and the NCR Medical Directorate for fiscal years 2009 through 2013.

We conducted this performance audit from May 2014 to January 2015 in accordance with generally accepted government auditing standards. Those standards require that we plan and perform the audit to obtain sufficient, appropriate evidence to provide a reasonable basis for our findings and conclusions based on our audit objectives. We believe that the evidence obtained provides a reasonable basis for our findings and conclusions based on our audit objectives.

BACKGROUND

The MHS operated by DOD has two missions: (1) supporting wartime and other deployments and (2) providing peacetime health care.[10] In support of these two missions, DOD operates a large and complex health care system that employs more than 150,000 military, civilian, and contract personnel working in military medical facilities, commonly referred to as military treatment facilities (MTF).

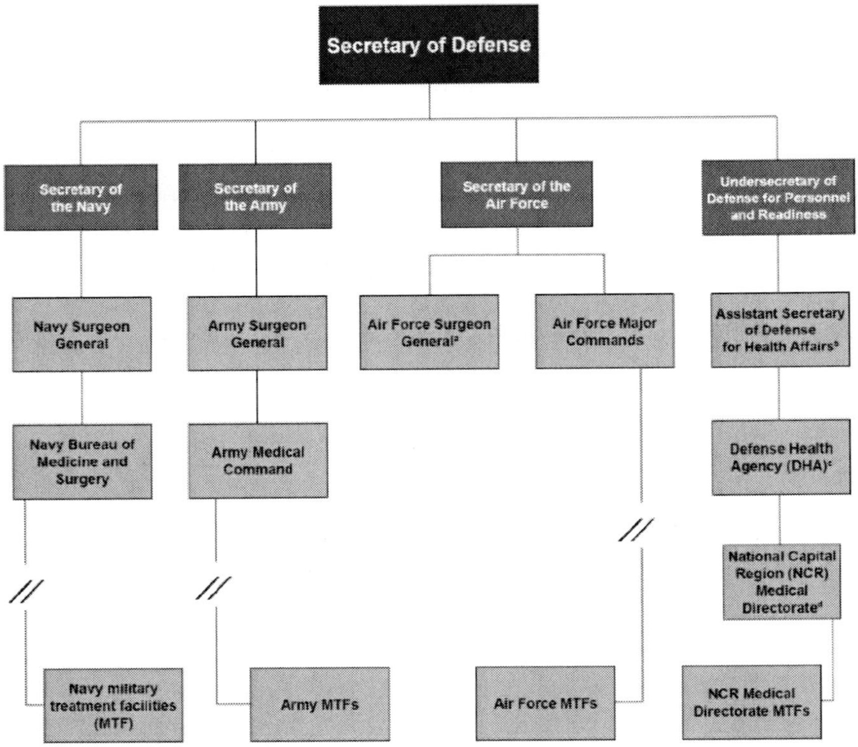

Source: GAO. | GAO-15-184.

[a]The Air Force Surgeon General does not have direct authority over Air Force MTFs; however, the Air Force Surgeon General exercises similar authority to that of the other Surgeons General through his role as medical advisor to the Air Force Chief of Staff.

[b]The Assistant Secretary of Defense for Health Affairs is the principal advisor for all DOD health policies and programs. The Office of the Assistant Secretary of Defense for Health Affairs (OASD HA) also has the authority to issue DOD instructions, publications, and memorandums that implement policy approved by the Secretary of Defense or the Under Secretary of Defense for Personnel and Readiness.

[c]DHA was established to support greater integration of clinical and business processes across the MHS. DHA manages the execution of policies issued by OASD HA, oversees the TRICARE health plan, and also exercises authority and control over the MTFs and subordinate clinics assigned to the NCR Medical Directorate.

[d]The NCR Medical Directorate was initially established as a DOD joint task force in September 2007 to operate DOD's medical facilities in the national capital region—including Walter Reed National Military Medical Center, Fort Belvoir Community Hospital, and their supporting clinics.

The NCR Medical Directorate reassigned civilian personnel from the military services to the NCR Medical Directorate, while retaining military health care providers within the appropriate military service's command and control.

Figure 1. Governance Structure of the Department of Defense (DOD) Military Health System (MHS).

In terms of the MHS organization and structure, OASD HA serves as the principal advisor for all DOD health policies and programs. OASD HA has the authority to issue DOD instructions, publications, and memorandums that implement policy approved by the Secretary of Defense or the Under Secretary of Defense for Personnel and Readiness and govern the management of DOD medical programs. In October 2013, the Defense Health Agency (DHA) was established to support greater integration of clinical and business processes across the MHS. The DHA manages the execution of policies issued by OASD HA, oversees the TRICARE health plan, and also exercises authority and control over the MTFs and subordinate clinics assigned to the NCR Medical Directorate.[11]

MTFs and their subordinate clinics are operated by either a military service or the NCR Medical Directorate. Neither OASD HA nor DHA have direct command and control of MTFs operated solely by the military services.[12] Each military service recruits, trains, and funds its own medical personnel to administer medical programs and provide medical services to beneficiaries. The NCR Medical Directorate has direct authority over civilian providers and personnel working within its facilities; however, the military services maintain authority over all military providers and personnel working within NCR Medical Directorate MTFs. See figure 1 for the current organizational and governance structure of the MHS.

DOD and the Military Services Have Increased the Number of Mental Health Providers to About 6,200—An Increase of Over a Third between Fiscal Years 2009 and 2013

The MHS has increased its overall mental health provider staffing level by 34 percent between fiscal years 2009 and 2013. Specifically, DOD increased the number of providers across the MHS from 4,608 providers in fiscal year 2009 to 6,186 providers in fiscal year 2013.[13] (See app. I for more information on fiscal year 2013 mental health provider staffing.) This increase was in response to a requirement in the NDAA for Fiscal Year 2010 that DOD increase its mental health capabilities.[14] (See app. II for more information on the recruitment and retention of DOD mental health providers.)

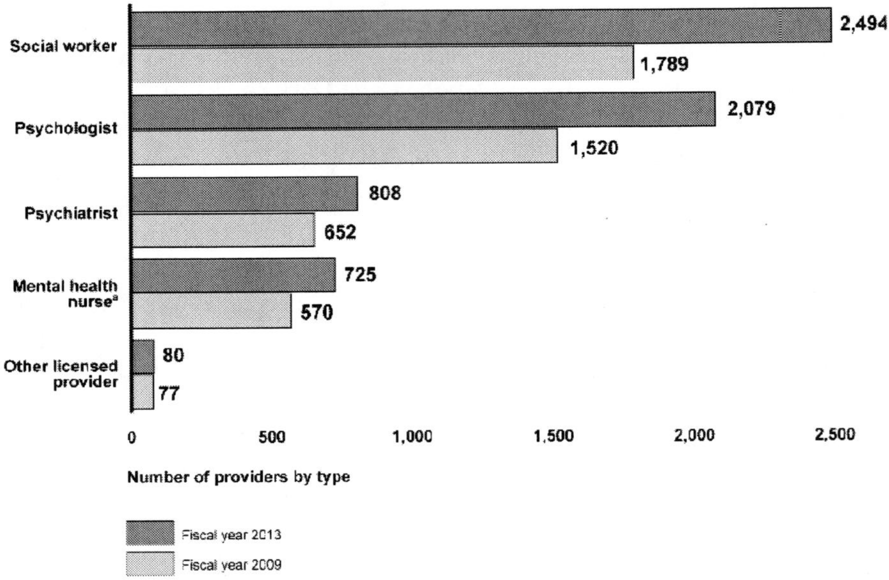

Source: GAO analysis of DOD data. | GAO-15-184.

Notes: The total number of DOD mental health providers in fiscal year 2013 was 6,186. The total number of DOD mental health providers in fiscal year 2009 was 4,608. Mental health provider totals in this figure have been rounded to the nearest full-time equivalent.

[a]The mental health nurse category includes both mental health nurse practitioners and mental health registered nurses. In fiscal year 2009, DOD did not report separate employment information on these two types of mental health providers.

Figure 2. Total Department of Defense (DOD) Mental Health Providers by Provider Type, September 2009 Compared to September 2013.

The type of mental health providers added to the MHS from fiscal year 2009 to fiscal year 2013 varied. (See fig. 2.) Specifically, social workers and psychologists were the most frequently added types of mental health providers during this period, while psychiatrists and mental health nurses were the least frequently added. The Army drove the overall increase in social workers and psychologists by adding 496 of the 705 social workers and 421 of the 559 psychologists to the MHS during this period. The Air Force added more social workers (64) than any other type of provider during this period, while the Navy added more psychologists (32) and other licensed providers (32). (See app. III for additional information on the breakdown of mental health provider staffing level changes for each military service from fiscal year 2009 to fiscal year 2013.)

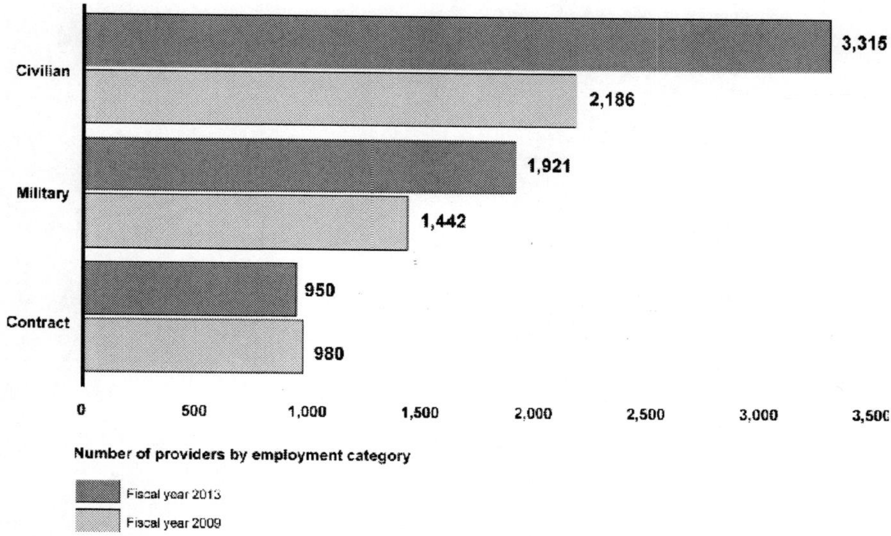

Source: GAO analysis of DOD data. | GAO-15-184.

Notes: The total number of DOD mental health providers for fiscal year 2013 was 6,186. The total number of DOD mental health providers for fiscal year 2009 was 4,608. Mental health provider totals in this figure have been rounded to the nearest full-time equivalent.

Figure 3. Total Department of Defense (DOD) Mental Health Providers by Employment Category, September 2009 Compared to September 2013.

During this time frame, the composition of DOD mental health provider staff by employment category also changed. Across the MHS, the number of civilian mental health providers increased by 52 percent (1,129) and military mental health providers increased by 33 percent (479), while the number of contract mental health providers decreased by 3 percent (30). (See fig. 3.) The services' individual changes varied, with the Army driving this systemic shift to civilian providers. Specifically, the Army added 863 new civilian mental health providers (a 50 percent increase), while decreasing the number of contract mental health providers by 153 (a 33 percent decrease). The Air Force also increased its civilian mental health provider staffing by 5 providers (a 2 percent increase) and increased its contract mental health provider staffing by 72 providers (a 39 percent increase). The Navy increased its number of military mental health providers by 113 (a 38 percent increase), added 12 civilian mental health providers (a 5 percent increase), and decreased contract mental health providers by 37 (an 11 percent decrease).

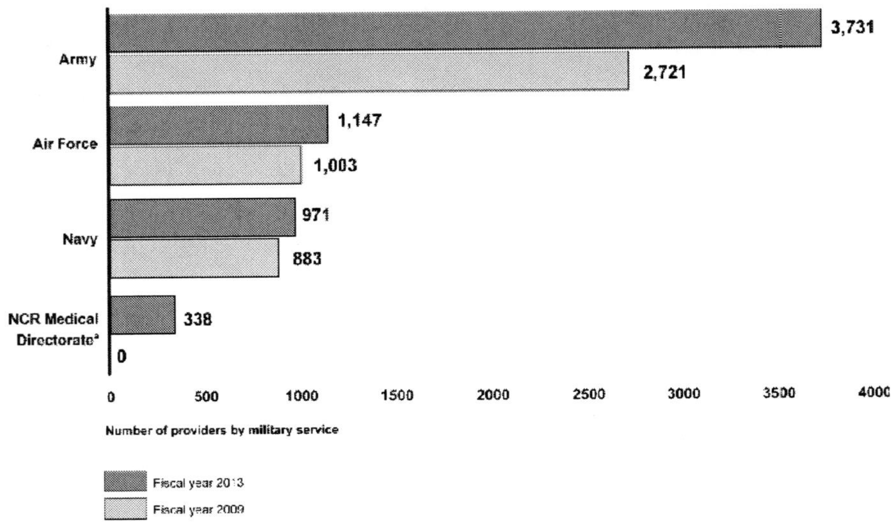

Source: GAO analysis of DOD data. | GAO-15-184.

Notes: The total number of DOD mental health providers in fiscal year 2013 was 6,186. The total number of DOD mental health providers in fiscal year 2009 was 4,608. Mental health provider totals in this figure have been rounded to the nearest full-time equivalent.

[a]In fiscal year 2009, all civilian and contract mental health providers assigned to the military treatment facilities (MTF) and subordinate clinics that are now within the NCR Medical Directorate were included in the military service totals, because at that time all MTFs within the NCR Medical Directorate were managed by multiple military services. In fiscal year 2013, the NCR Medical Directorate reported its own civilian and contract mental health provider totals while retaining military mental health providers within the appropriate military services' figures.

Figure 4. Total Department of Defense (DOD) Mental Health Providers by Military Service and the National Capital Region (NCR) Medical Directorate, September 2009 Compared to September 2013.

While all three military services increased their mental health provider staffing from fiscal year 2009 to fiscal year 2013, the Army's addition of

1,010 mental health providers represented the largest portion of the DOD-wide increase. The Navy's increase of 88 mental health providers was the smallest portion of the DOD-wide increase. (See fig. 4.)

DOD CREATED A MODEL FOR DEVELOPING MENTAL HEALTH PROVIDER STAFFING NEEDS, BUT THE MILITARY SERVICES DO NOT USE IT CONSISTENTLY

DOD created the Psychological Health Risk-Adjusted Model for Staffing (PHRAMS) to show current and estimate future mental health provider staffing needs of the MHS. In fiscal year 2014, PHRAMS was used for a common purpose by the military services for the first time—the development of the fiscal year 2016 DOD budget request for mental health programs.[15] However, the military services are either not using PHRAMS as the primary basis of their estimates of mental health provider staffing needs or supplementing their PHRAMS results with service-specific staffing methods. This limits DOD's ability to consistently assess mental health provider staffing needs throughout the MHS.

DOD Created PHRAMS to Estimate Its Current and Future Mental Health Provider Staffing Needs

PHRAMS projects the number and mix of providers needed to meet the mental health care needs of the MHS. In fiscal year 2007, DOD contracted with a non-profit research and analysis organization to develop PHRAMS in response to recommendations from the DOD Task Force on Mental Health.[16] These recommendations included that: (1) Congress fund and DOD allocate sufficient staff to provide a full continuum of mental health services to servicemembers and their dependents and (2) DOD adopt a risk-adjusted population-based model to calculate mental health staffing needs. As of September 2014, the contract to develop and maintain PHRAMS had cost DOD $2 million, according to DOD officials.

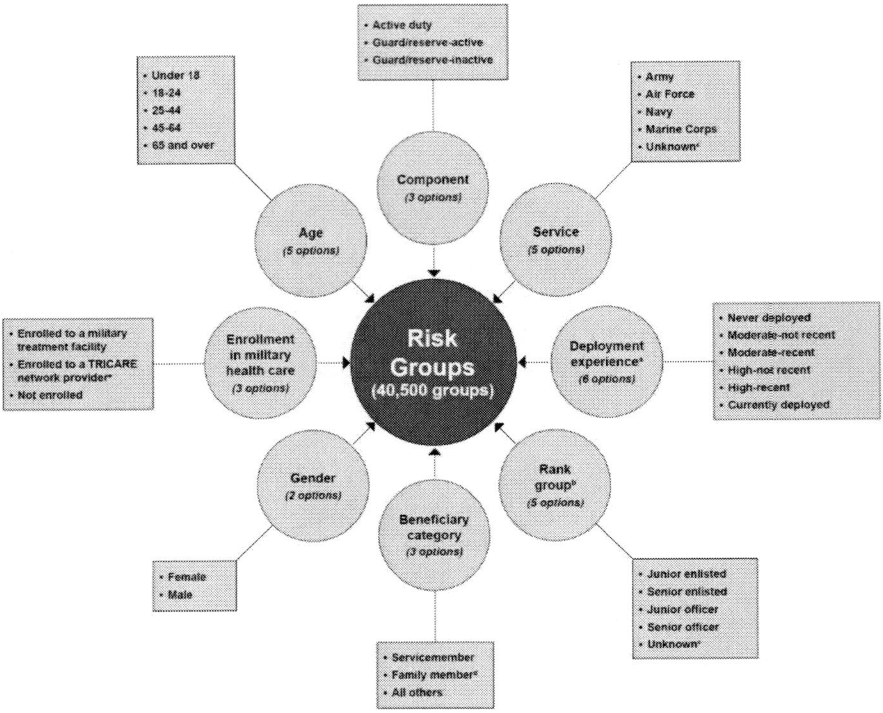

Source: GAO analysis of DOD data. | GAO-15-184.

Notes: This figure includes all risk factors included in version 5 of PHRAMS.

[a]Deployment experience is a combination of how recently servicemembers have been deployed and the degree of their deployments. PHRAMS considers servicemembers to be recently deployed if they deployed within the past year. The degree of deployment is a combination of the number of deployments and the cumulative number of months a servicemember has been deployed between September 2001 and the end of fiscal year 2012. Servicemembers will have high degrees of deployment if one of two conditions occur: (1) they have been cumulatively deployed for 12 months or more or (2) they have been cumulatively deployed for 6 to 12 months with fewer than 3 deployments. Servicemembers have moderate degrees of deployment if they have ever deployed and do not meet the criteria for a high degree of deployment.

[b]Rank groups are divided into junior and senior categories. For enlisted servicemembers, the first four ranks in each military service are considered junior and the next five ranks are considered senior. For officers, the first three ranks in each military service are considered junior and the next seven ranks are considered senior. Warrant Officers are categorized as senior enlisted.

[c] A small percentage of the beneficiary population has missing information for one or more risk factor data elements. PHRAMS assigns these individuals to an "unknown" group.

[d] Risk factor values for component, service, deployment experience, and rank group for family members are populated using the sponsoring servicemember's information.

[e] In addition to operating its own health care facilities, DOD also provides health care to servicemembers, dependents, and military retirees through its TRICARE purchased care network. TRICARE supplements the health care resources of DOD with networks of civilian health care providers.

Figure 5. Risk Factors Included in the Department of Defense (DOD) Psychological Health Risk-Adjusted Model for Staffing (PHRAMS).

PHRAMS is designed to be a common DOD-wide model that can be used by the military services to assess current mental health provider staffing needs and forecast these staffing needs over a 5-year timeframe.[17] DOD intended PHRAMS to allow the Department to fulfill two goals: (1) assess whether or not there are enough mental health providers within the MHS to meet the increased mental health needs of servicemembers and their dependents that resulted from their experiences in recent conflicts, and (2) allow the Department to report the mental health provider staffing needs of the MHS to Congress. DHA and the PHRAMS contractor engage in an annual model review process to incorporate changes requested by the military services into the next version of the model. According to DHA officials, PHRAMS was used for a common purpose for the first time in fiscal year 2014—the development of the DOD fiscal year 2016 budget request for mental health programs.

To assess current mental health provider staffing needs and determine 5-year forecasts of these needs, PHRAMS places MHS beneficiaries— including servicemembers, dependents, and other beneficiaries—into 40,500 individual risk groups based on unique combinations of eight risk factors. [18] (See fig. 5.)

To determine MTF-based mental health provider staffing needs,[19] PHRAMS calculates three key aspects of mental health services in the MHS—(1) the beneficiary demand for mental health services; (2) the number of appointments needed to treat these conditions, referred to as encounters; and (3) the availability of MHS mental health providers to supply these encounters. (See fig. 6.)

- **Beneficiary demand for mental health services**. PHRAMS uses historical data to determine the prevalence of certain mental health diagnoses within each of the 40,500 risk groups included in the model.[20] These prevalence rates are then combined with projections of the number of beneficiaries in each risk group to estimate the demand for mental health services each risk group will place on the MHS.[21]

- **Number of appointments (encounter rate)**. PHRAMS calculates the number of appointments that will be needed to treat diagnosed beneficiaries within each risk group. To do this, the model applies predetermined encounter rates that specify how many times a beneficiary with each mental health diagnosis included in the model will interact with an MTF provider.[22]
- **Availability of MHS mental health providers**. PHRAMS then determines the number of encounters each MTF-based mental health provider can supply each year by multiplying the number of encounters that can be completed each hour (encounter time) by the total number of annual hours each mental health provider can spend supplying mental health services to beneficiaries (provider time).[23]

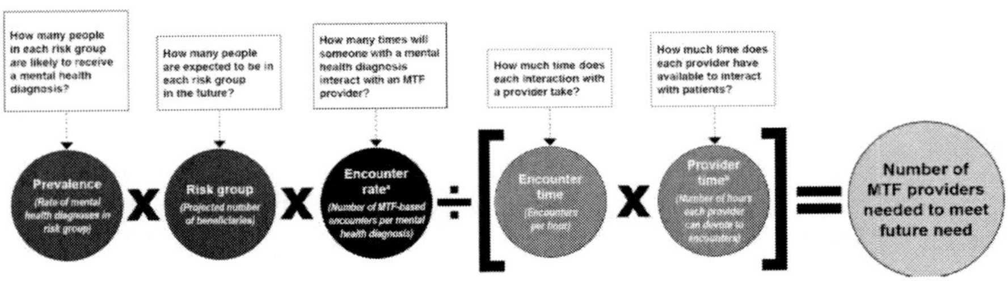

Source: GAO analysis of DOD data. | GAO-15-184.

Notes: This figure includes information from version 5 of PHRAMS. PHRAMS is also used to estimate the number of TRICARE providers that will be needed to provide mental health services to beneficiaries enrolled in the TRICARE network.

[a]To establish the encounter rates used in PHRAMS, the PHRAMS contractor created a composite encounter rate for each mental health condition included in the model based on five inputs: (1) recommendations from a Navy work group, (2) recommendations from an Air Force work group, (3) information gathered from reviews of clinical literature, (4) information gathered from reviews of clinical practice guidelines, and (5) other interviews. Encounter rates are also adjusted based on historical data. PHRAMS assigns all predicted encounters to either MTFs or the TRICARE network. Within the model, military service users can modify the percentage of encounters that are assigned to MTFs and the TRICARE network.

[b]Military and civilian mental health providers have different amounts of hours they can devote to encounters each year. For example, the default value in PHRAMS version 5 for military mental health providers' clinical encounter time was set at

1,190 hours per year, while the default value for civilian mental health providers' clinical encounter time was set at 1,399.
This difference accounts for the hours military mental health providers spend each year performing military-specific duties not related to beneficiary care and differences in assumed productivity for military and civilian mental health care providers.

Figure 6. Department of Defense (DOD) Psychological Health Risk-Adjusted Model for Staffing (PHRAMS) Military Treatment Facility (MTF)-Based Mental Health Provider Needs Calculation.

Military Services Mental Health Provider Estimates Are Not Based Mainly on PHRAMS

Despite all military services agreeing to use PHRAMS to generate their estimates of mental health provider staffing needs for the fiscal year 2016 budget request, the military services either did not use PHRAMS as the main basis for their mental health provider staffing estimates or supplemented PHRAMS results using other service-specific methods prior to submitting their fiscal year 2016 budget requests.[24] Standards for internal control in the federal government state that agencies' control activities should ensure that management's directives are carried out.[25] The military services reported making these adjustments because PHRAMS does not account for several factors that are crucial to their assessment of mental health provider staffing needs, specifically the following:

- **Army**. Army officials reported that they did not use PHRAMS as the basis for their fiscal year 2016 budget request and instead determined their mental health provider staffing needs through their legacy staffing model and adjusted PHRAMS to ensure it produced similar results. Unlike PHRAMS, which bases its mental health provider staffing estimates on beneficiary demand for services, the Army legacy staffing model uses historical workload data to estimate future staffing needs in multiple specialties, including mental health.[26] The Army legacy staffing model uses projected beneficiary population changes to adjust the historical workload for Army MTFs up or down as needed. According to the Army official responsible for generating manpower estimates for Army MTFs, PHRAMS does not currently meet the needs of the Army. This is because PHRAMS' assumption that all military services experience the same encounter rates for mental health conditions included in the model is an overgeneralization of mental health service demands. This official believes that this is particularly problematic for the Army because deployments are more traumatic for Army servicemembers and may result in some servicemembers requiring more than the average number of encounters. As a result, the Army only ran PHRAMS after the military service had already determined its mental health provider staffing needs through its legacy staffing model.

- **Air Force**. According to Air Force officials, while the Air Force uses some aspects of PHRAMS, it did not rely exclusively on PHRAMS to generate their estimates of mental health staffing needs included in the fiscal year 2016 budget request. These officials explained that PHRAMS was the first step in a three-step process used to generate the Air Force's fiscal year 2016 budget request for mental health provider staffing. First, Air Force manpower staff ran PHRAMS and provided the PHRAMS-generated mental health provider staffing estimates to Air Force's mental health consultants for consideration.[27] Second, the Air Force mental health consultants developed multiple staffing level proposals by combining the PHRAMS output with their own expertise and information received during conversations with Air Force MTF officials. Finally, the Chief of Clinical Operations for the Air Force Medical Support Agency selected the best staffing proposal among those submitted for review by the Air Force mental health consultants. Air Force officials reported that this process was applied because PHRAMS relies on data that is several years old and does not take into account all aspects of Air Force mental health provider staffing, such as mental health providers embedded in operational units. Air Force officials also explained that they plan to continue using this process in the future to generate mental health provider staffing estimates.
- **Navy**. Navy officials reported that they used PHRAMS, but supplemented PHRAMS estimates of mental health provider staffing needs with additional information. According to Navy officials, this was necessary because PHRAMS does not include estimates of mental health provider staffing needs on Navy vessels and for deployed Marine Corps units. As a result, Navy officials adjusted their PHRAMS output to account for these additional needs for mental health providers. These officials explained that they relied on

traditional methods—such as on-site industrial engineering reviews and industry standards—to calculate these operational requirements for Navy mental health providers. According to Navy officials, the fiscal year 2016 budget request submitted by the Navy for mental health provider staffing is the sum of the estimated staffing levels generated by PHRAMS and the calculated operational requirements for mental health providers.

When we shared this information with DHA officials, they told us that they were unaware of specific supplemental or alternative methods used by the military services to determine their final mental health provider staffing estimates. However, these officials did note that the military services do make modifications to their PHRAMS results through modifying certain aspects of the model and DHA does not collect information on these modifications. DHA and the PHRAMS contractor review the model annually to incorporate changes requested by the military services in the next version of the model. Standards for internal control in the federal government state that information should be recorded and communicated to management and others within the agency that need it in a format and time frame that enables them to carry out their responsibilities.[28] However, since DHA did not have access to this information on how the military services supplemented PHRAMS for their fiscal year 2016 budget request, this critical information was not included in this annual update process.

As a result of the military services' alterations to PHRAMS estimates of mental health provider staffing needs, DHA cannot consistently determine how beneficiary demand affects the mental health provider staffing needs for the MHS.

Specifically, due to the Army's use of a workload-based staffing estimate, the resulting mental health provider staffing needs estimates submitted for the fiscal year 2016 budget process may not consistently reflect the beneficiary demand for mental health services across military services. In addition, without an accurate picture of the ways the military services altered or supplemented PHRAMS results, DHA cannot evaluate the role PHRAMS played in the development of the fiscal year 2016 budget request for mental health provider staffing and cannot ensure that it is directing the PHRAMS contractor to make the most appropriate changes to the model that minimize the need for these service-specific supplements.

Military Services Report Mental Health Provider Staffing Levels on Quarterly Reports Submitted to DHA, But Do Not Report Reliable Information on Future Needs

The military services submit quarterly reports to DHA through the OASD HA human capital office that include information on their current mental health provider staffing levels and should, as requested, include information on their future needs for these providers. However, the military services do not include reliable information about their mental health provider staffing needs on these quarterly reports, despite having access to PHRAMS since fiscal year 2010.[29] As a result, DHA does not have an accurate picture of the mental health provider staffing needs of the MHS and cannot accurately report this information to Congress. Standards for internal control in the federal government state that information should be recorded and communicated to management and others within the agency that need it in a format and time frame that enables them to carry out their responsibilities.[30]

DHA requests information each quarter from the military services and the NCR Medical Directorate on mental health provider staffing in order to understand the MHS-wide use and need for these providers and report this information to Congress when requested. Each military service and the NCR Medical Directorate submits quarterly staffing reports to DHA through the OASD HA human capital office that include information on three areas of mental health provider staffing: (1) the number of mental health providers each military service needs to fulfill the needs of their beneficiaries, referred to as requirements; (2) the number of authorized positions each military service has for various types of mental health providers, referred to as authorizations; and (3) the actual number of mental health providers each military service has working within their MTFs and subordinate clinics that quarter, referred to as on-board providers. However, we found that information reported is unreliable. Specifically, we found the following:

- According to DHA officials, only the Army submits information on the number of mental health providers its MTFs and subordinate clinics need to serve Army beneficiaries and it derives these numbers from the Army workload-based legacy staffing model.
- DHA officials told us that the Navy and the Air Force do not track needs for mental health provider staffing. Instead, they submit the

number of authorized mental health provider positions for both the requirements and authorizations sections of these quarterly reports. NCR Medical Directorate officials told us that the requirements section of their quarterly reports are populated using the staffing needs identified in the intermediate manpower planning documents that were created during the formation of the NCR Medical Directorate. According to DOD officials, the NCR Medical Directorate is currently reviewing the staffing needs of its MTFs and subordinate clinics and anticipates completion of this review by December 2014.

Without reliable information from the military services and the NCR Medical Directorate on the quarterly reports, DHA cannot assess the need for mental health providers throughout the MHS and cannot ensure that it is providing assistance to the military services in meeting their unmet needs. The military services have had access to PHRAMS since fiscal year 2010 and the model could be used to assess the mental health provider needs of each military service and the NCR Medical Directorate on an ongoing basis. Incorporating this information into the requirements section of the quarterly reports each military service and the NCR Medical Directorate submit to DHA through the OASD HA human capital office would provide this important information to DHA. In addition, this information would also ensure greater consistency in the military services' and the NCR Medical Directorate's assessment of this aspect of mental health provider staffing and ensure greater accuracy in DOD's reports to Congress about mental health provider staffing.

CONCLUSION

While PHRAMS has been in development since fiscal year 2007, the military services only recently began using the model for a common purpose—the fiscal year 2016 DOD budget request. However, PHRAMS is not meeting its intended goals because the military services are not using it consistently to assess their mental health provider staffing needs. Instead, the military services are supplementing PHRAMS mental health provider staffing estimates with additional information. It is critical that the military services report how they have supplemented PHRAMS to ensure (1) that DHA and the PHRAMS contractor can correctly analyze and interpret the military services' mental health provider staffing estimates, and (2) that PHRAMS is updated regularly to meet the needs of the military services. DHA is also unable to generate accurate reports to Congress on the staffing needs of the entire MHS, because the military services are not using PHRAMS to generate consistent mental health provider staffing needs estimates and are instead reporting unreliable estimates on their quarterly reports. DHA is therefore unable to assess and report on current mental health provider staffing needs.

RECOMMENDATIONS FOR EXECUTIVE ACTION

To ensure DHA can accurately and consistently assess mental health provider staffing needs across each of the military services, we recommend that the Secretary of Defense direct the Secretaries of the Army, Air Force, and Navy to take the following two actions:

- Require the medical commands of each military service to report any additional service-specific methods they use to determine their final estimates of mental health provider staffing needs; and
- Require the medical commands of each military service to include its estimated mental health provider staffing needs generated through PHRAMS in the requirements fields of DHA's quarterly mental health staffing reports.

We further recommend that the Secretary of Defense direct the Assistant Secretary of Defense for Health Affairs to take the following two actions:

- Ensure DHA, through the PHRAMS contractor, continue to refine PHRAMS to incorporate the needs of the military services to reduce the need for additional service-specific methods of determining mental health provider staffing needs; and
- Require the NCR Medical Directorate to include its estimated mental health provider staffing needs generated through PHRAMS in the requirements fields of DHA's quarterly mental health staffing reports.

AGENCY COMMENTS AND OUR EVALUATION

In its comments, DOD generally concurred with two of our four recommendations. DOD also provided technical comments, which we have incorporated as appropriate.

DOD concurred with our recommendation that the Secretary of Defense should direct the Secretaries of the Army, the Air Force, and the Navy to require the medical commands of each military service to report any additional service-specific methods they use to determine their final estimates of mental health provider staffing needs. DOD did not provide a time frame or action plan for implementing this recommendation.

In addition, in response to our recommendation that the Secretary of Defense ensure DHA, through the PHRAMS contractor, continue to refine PHRAMS to incorporate the needs of military services to reduce the need for additional service-specific methods of determining mental health provider staffing needs, DOD said that DHA continues to serve in an advisory role to the military services to ensure that the next version of PHRAMS meets each service's needs. DOD did not provide a time frame or action plan for implementing this recommendation.

DOD did not concur with our recommendations to require the medical commands of each military service and the NCR Medical Directorate to include their estimated mental health provider staffing needs generated through PHRAMS in the requirements field of DHA's quarterly mental health staffing reports. DOD stated in its comments that using PHRAMS in the requirements fields of these reports will not add value to the quarterly mental health staffing reports and noted that the military services do not use PHRAMS as the sole source of mental health requirements. We disagree with DOD's conclusion and maintain that our recommendations should be implemented.

The military services and the NCR Medical Directorate are not currently providing DHA with consistent information that it can rely on to: (1) make informed decisions regarding the MHS-wide usage and need for mental health providers and (2) develop reports to Congress based on this information.

Specifically, only one military service—the Army—reports the number of mental health providers that its MTFs need to serve Army beneficiaries in the requirements field of DHA's quarterly mental health staffing reports. The other two military services—the Air Force and the Navy—enter the number of mental health providers that were authorized by DOD for that fiscal year in the requirements field because they do not track mental health provider staffing needs.

Additionally, the NCR Medical Directorate told us that it populates the requirements field of DHA's quarterly mental health staffing reports with information that was created during the formation of the NCR Medical Directorate several years ago and not with the current needs of its beneficiary population. We believe that to adequately assess the need for mental health providers throughout the MHS, DHA needs to have access to consistent and reliable information on mental health provider staffing needs in the quarterly mental health staffing reports. By not supplying consistent information on mental health provider staffing needs generated through PHRAMS—a common staffing model all military services and the NCR Medical Directorate have access to—the military services and the NCR Medical Directorate make it difficult to properly assess relative mental health provider staffing needs across the services. If our recommendations were implemented, DHA would have access to consistent information about mental health provider staffing needs throughout the MHS and would be able to more reliably report this information to Congress.

Randall B. Williamson
Director, Health Care

APPENDIX I: FISCAL YEAR 2013 DEPARTMENT OF DEFENSE MENTAL HEALTH PROVIDER STAFFING

This appendix provides results from our analysis of Department of Defense (DOD) fiscal year 2013 quarterly mental health staffing reports. Each military service and the National Capital Region (NCR) Medical Directorate submit these reports to the Defense Health Agency (DHA) through the Office of the Assistant Secretary of Defense for Health Affairs (OASD HA) human capital office each quarter to identify their mental health staffing levels and needs.

- Figure 7 shows the total number of mental health providers working within the MHS by provider type as of September 2013.
- Figure 8 shows the total number of mental health providers working within the MHS by employment category as of September 2013.[1]

- Figure 9 shows the total number of mental health providers working within the MHS by military service and the NCR Medical Directorate as of September 2013.
- Table 1 shows the mental health provider staffing levels for the Army as of September 2013.
- Table 2 shows the mental health provider staffing levels for the Air Force as of September 2013.
- Table 3 shows the mental health provider staffing levels for the Navy as of September 2013.
- Table 4 shows the mental health provider staffing levels for the NCR Medical Directorate as of September 2013.

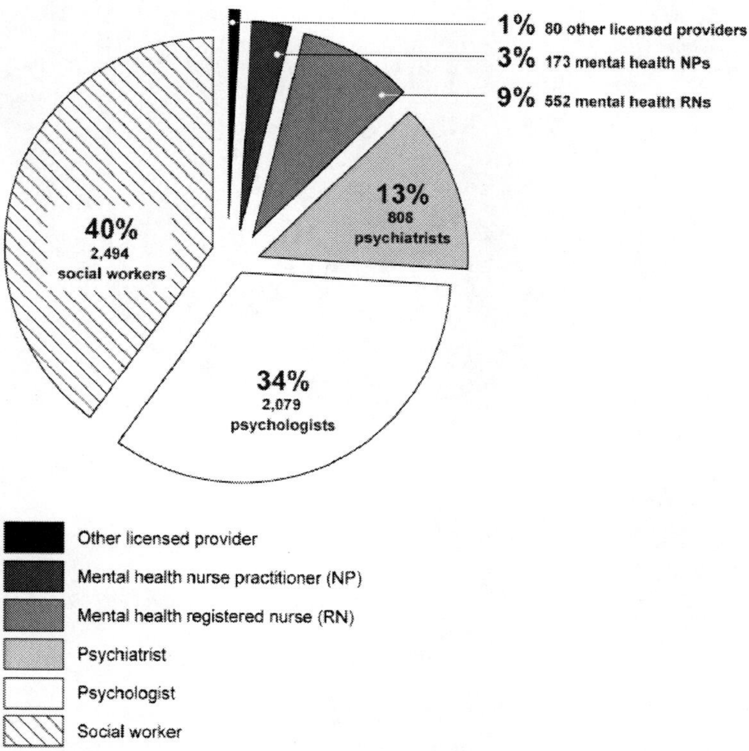

Source: GAO analysis of DOD data. I GAO-15-184.

Note: The total number of DOD mental health providers in fiscal year 2013 was 6,186. Mental health provider totals and percentages in this figure have been rounded to the nearest full-time equivalent.

Figure 7. Total Department of Defense (DOD) Mental Health Providers by Provider Type, September 2013.

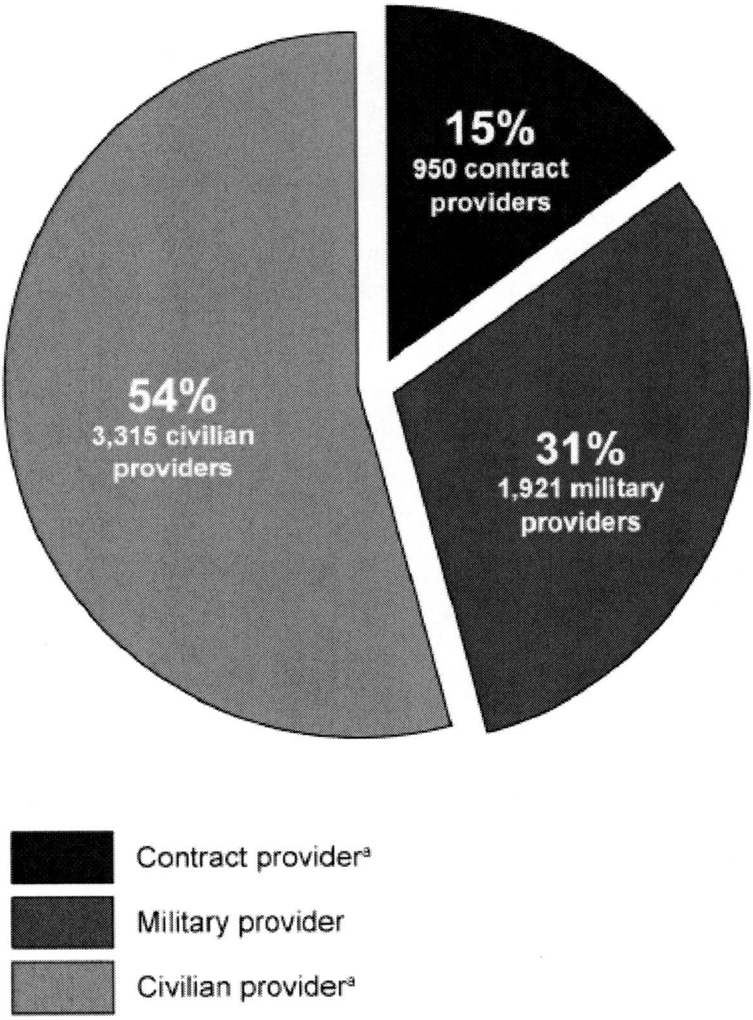

Source: GAO analysis of DOD data. I GAO-15-184.

Note: The total number of DOD mental health providers in fiscal year 2013 was 6,186. Mental health provider totals and percentages in this figure have been rounded to the nearest full-time equivalent.

[a] Civilian and contract providers are represented as full-time employee equivalent positions.

Figure 8. Total Department of Defense (DOD) Mental Health Providers by Employment Category, September 2013.

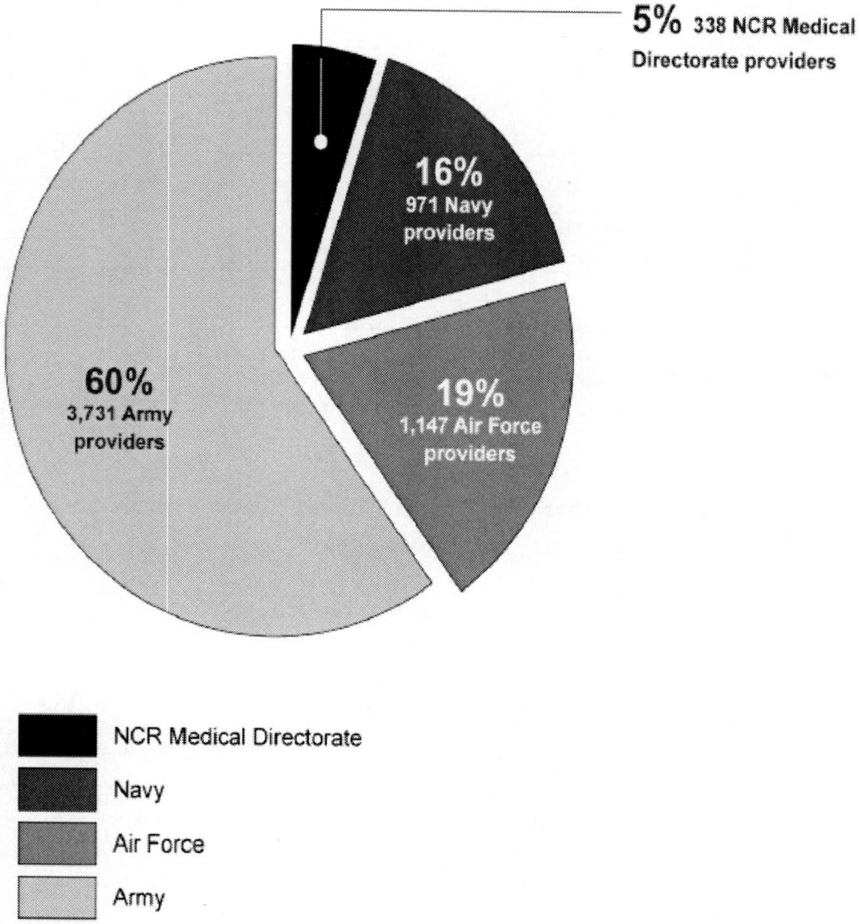

Source: GAO analysis of DOD data. | GAO-15-184.

Note: The total number of DOD mental health providers in fiscal year 2013 was 6,186. Mental health provider totals and percentages in this figure have been rounded to the nearest full-time equivalent.

Figure 9. Total Department of Defense (DOD) Mental Health Providers by Military Service and the National Capital Region (NCR) Medical Directorate, September 2013.

Table 1. Total Number of Army Mental Health Providers as of September 2013

Provider type	Employment category			Total
	Military	Civilian	Contract	
Psychiatrist	199	140	91	430
Psychologist	239	980	78	1,297
Mental health nurse practitioner	37	47	20	104
Mental health registered nurse	91	117	13	221
Social worker	273	1,298	107	1,678
Other licensed provider	0	0	0	0
Total	**839**	**2,582**	**310**[a]	**3,731**[a]

Source: GAO analysis of Department of Defense data. | GAO-15-184.

[a]Numbers do not total due to rounding to the nearest number of full-time equivalent positions.

Table 2. Total Number of Air Force Mental Health Providers as of September 2013

Provider type	Employment category			Total
	Military	Civilian	Contract	
Psychiatrist	132	5	9	**146**
Psychologist	247	14	103	**364**
Mental health nurse practitioner	26	0	0	**26**
Mental health registered nurse	39	53	28	**120**
Social worker	231	143	117	**491**
Other licensed provider	0	0	0	**0**
Total	**675**	**215**	**257**	**1,147**

Source: GAO analysis of Department of Defense data. | GAO-15-184.

Table 3. Total Number of Navy Mental Health Providers as of September 2013

Provider type	Employment category			Total
	Military	Civilian	Contract	
Psychiatrist	109	38	28	175
Psychologist	144	103	93	340
Mental health nurse practitioner	32	2	9	43
Mental health registered nurse	71	14	68	153
Social worker	51	89	66	206
Other licensed provider	0	23	31	54
Total	**407**	**269**	**295**	**971**

Source: GAO analysis of Department of Defense data. | GAO-15-184.

Table 4. Total Number of National Capital Region (NCR) Medical Directorate Mental Health Providers as of September 2013

Provider type	Employment category			Total
	Military[a]	Civilian	Contract	
Psychiatrist	0	51	6	57
Psychologist	0	56	22	78
Mental health nurse practitioner	0	0	0	0
Mental health registered nurse	0	40	18	58
Social worker	0	86	33	119
Other licensed provider	0	16	10	26
Total	**0**	**249**	**89**	**338**

Source: GAO analysis of Department of Defense (DOD) data. | GAO-15-184.

[a]The NCR Medical Directorate was initially established as a DOD joint task force in September 2007 to operate DOD's medical facilities in the national capital region—including Walter Reed National Military Medical Center, Fort Belvoir Community Hospital, and supporting clinics. The NCR Medical Directorate reassigned civilian and contract personnel from the military services to the NCR Medical Directorate while retaining military mental health providers within the appropriate military services' figures.

Appendix II: Recruitment and Retention of Department of Defense Mental Health Providers

This appendix provides information on the recruitment and retention of Department of Defense (DOD) mental health providers. Specifically, we discuss (1) the mechanisms the military services use to recruit and retain mental health providers, and (2) the challenges the military services experience in recruiting and retaining mental health providers.

To determine the mechanisms the military services use to recruit and retain mental health providers, we reviewed relevant laws, including each National Defense Authorization Act (NDAA) from fiscal years 2010 through 2014, to determine the recruitment and retention mechanisms available to DOD for mental health providers. We also spoke with officials from Office of the Assistant Secretary of Defense for Health Affairs (OASD HA), Army, Air Force, and Navy about their use of these mechanisms.

To determine the challenges the military services experience in recruiting and retaining mental health providers, we spoke with officials from OASD HA, Army, Air Force, and Navy. We also reviewed the Health Resources and

Services Administration's Health Professional Shortage Area designations to determine whether other health care delivery systems also experienced challenges in recruiting and retaining certain mental health providers.[1]

Military Services Use Numerous Mechanisms to Recruit and Retain Mental Health Providers

All three military services reported using numerous recruitment and retention mechanisms, many of which are cited in the NDAA for Fiscal Year 2010. These mechanisms include the following:[2]

- **Health Professions Scholarship and Financial Assistance Program (HPSP)**. Officials from all three military services reported using this program to recruit various types of medical providers, including mental health providers. Through HPSP, the military services provide scholarships, stipends, and other benefits for students in advanced health care fields—including physicians, psychiatric nurse practitioners, and psychologists.[3] The military services reported that HPSP was a particularly important recruitment tool for physicians, including psychiatrists. However, officials from all three military services stressed that they cannot predict the exact number of psychiatrists HPSP will produce annually because it begins funding medical students' general training prior to their selection of a specialty.
- **Uniformed Services University of the Health Sciences (USUHS)**. All three military services reported that USUHS was a mechanism for recruiting and training clinical psychologists. USUHS trains, educates, and prepares military health providers, including clinical psychologists, to work in the military health system (MHS). 4 Officials from the military services reported that the annual enrollment in USUHS for clinical psychology students by service is Army, three students; Air Force, two to three students; and Navy, five students.
- **Bonuses for mental health providers**. Officials from all three military services reported using a variety of bonuses for mental health providers.[5] Specifically, the Army reported using accession, relocation, and retention bonuses for both military and civilian mental health providers. The Air Force reported that they provide accession

bonuses to fully-qualified military mental health providers, as well as bonuses for specialty board certification and a retention bonus after providers have completed a specified number of years-of-service. Finally, the Navy reported that all mental health specialties are eligible for some combination of accession and retention bonuses and board certification pay.

- **Direct-hire authority for civilian mental health providers**. Both the Army and Navy reported using direct-hire authority to recruit civilian mental health providers. The Office of Personnel Management can grant direct-hire authority to executive branch agencies to fill vacancies when a critical hiring need or severe shortage of candidates exists. Direct-hire authorities expedite hiring by eliminating some competitive hiring procedures, such as rating and ranking candidates, that would otherwise be required. Agencies may also pursue agency-specific direct-hire authorities.
- **Training program for licensed clinical social workers**. Both the Army and Navy reported using the Army's training program for licensed clinical social workers. In 2008, the Army created a program for training licensed clinical social workers with Fayetteville State University to address a shortage of Army social work military providers. This program provides participants with a Masters in Social Work and internship placements. The program annually trains up to 30 Army social work military providers, 5 Army National Guard social work military providers, and 2 Navy social work military providers.[6] Army officials reported that this program is satisfying all of its need for social work military providers annually, and Navy officials told us that this program was an important recruitment tool for their social work military providers as well.

Military Services Experience Several Challenges Recruiting and Retaining Mental Health Providers

In the face of nationwide shortages of mental health professionals, the ability to recruit and retain mental health providers, particularly psychiatrists, poses a challenge according to officials from all three military services. The Health Resources and Services Administration has reported nationwide shortages of psychiatrists and identified 3,900 health professional shortage areas throughout the nation with a relative scarcity of psychiatrists.[7] As of

January 2014, the Health Resources and Services Administration reported that it would take approximately 2,600 additional psychiatrists nationwide to eliminate the current shortages it has identified.

In addition to nationwide shortages of mental health professionals, there are other overarching military-specific challenges for all three military services as they compete for scarce mental health resources. Mental health provider recruitment and retention challenges specific to military service include:

- **Frequent deployments and relocations**. Officials from all three military services reported that both frequent deployments and relocations made it difficult for them to recruit and retain mental health military providers. For example, Navy officials told us that they have received feedback from psychiatrists leaving military service that requirements to move frequently and deploy were reasons they were leaving the Navy.
- **Assignment to work in remote locations**. According to officials from all three military services, the remote locations where many military treatment facilities are located posed recruitment and retention challenges for mental health providers. For example, Army officials explained that many Army bases are located relatively far away from major metropolitan areas and that mental health military, civilian, and contract providers are reluctant to be located in what they perceived to be remote and isolated locations for lengthy periods of time.
- **Competitive compensation for mental health providers**. Officials from all three military services reported that the inability of DOD to create compensation packages for civilian mental health providers, particularly psychiatrists, that were competitive with private sector compensation affected their ability to recruit and retain these providers. For example, Army officials stated that both a 3-year long DOD pay freeze and recent furloughs affected their ability to create competitive salaries for providers and contributed to the Army's 15 percent turnover rate in their psychiatrist and psychologist mental health provider populations in recent years.

APPENDIX III: MENTAL HEALTH PROVIDER STAFFING INCREASES BY MILITARY SERVICE

This appendix provides results from our analysis of Department of Defense (DOD) quarterly mental health staffing reports for fiscal years 2009 and 2013. Each service and the National Capital Region (NCR) Medical Directorate submits these reports to the Defense Health Agency (DHA) through the Office of the Assistant Secretary of Defense for Health Affairs (OASD HA) human capital office each quarter to identify their mental health staffing levels. The NCR Medical Directorate is not represented in this appendix because in fiscal year 2009 mental health provider staffing levels were included in the military service totals and, as a result, comparisons of NCR Medical Directorate staffing levels from fiscal year 2009 to fiscal year 2013 are not available.

- Table 5 provides results for mental health provider staffing levels for the Army in fiscal year 2009 and fiscal year 2013.
- Table 6 provides results for mental health provider staffing levels for the Air Force in fiscal year 2009 and fiscal year 2013.
- Table 7 provides results for mental health provider staffing levels for the Navy in fiscal year 2009 and fiscal year 2013.

Table 5. Total Number of Army Mental Health Providers, Fiscal Year 2009 Compared to Fiscal Year 2013

	Employment category							
	Military		Civilian		Contract		Total	
	Fiscal year		Fiscal year		Fiscal year		Fiscal year	
Provider type	2009	2013[a]	2009	2013[a]	2009	2013[a]	2009	2013[a]
Psychiatrist	126	199	118	140	92	91	336	430
Psychologist	187	239	579	980	110	78	876	1,297
Mental health nurse[b]	102	128	140	164	31	33	273	325
Social worker	125	273	882	1,298	175	107	1,182	1,678
Other licensed provider	0	0	0	0	55	0	55	0
Total	540	839	1,719	2,582	463	310[c]	2,721[c]	3,731[c]

Source: GAO analysis of Department of Defense (DOD) data. | GAO-15-184.

[a]Fiscal year 2013 values do not include civilian and contract providers assigned to military treatment facilities and subordinate clinics within the National Capital

Region Medical Directorate because beginning in fiscal year 2011 this command began reporting as a separate entity.

[b]The mental health nurse category includes both mental health nurse practitioners and mental health registered nurses. In fiscal year 2009, DOD did not report separate employment information on these two types of mental health providers.

[c]Numbers do not total due to rounding to the nearest number of full-time equivalent positions.

Table 6. Total Number of Air Force Mental Health Providers, Fiscal Year 2009 Compared to Fiscal Year 2013

	Employment category							
	Military		Civilian		Contract		Total	
	Fiscal year		Fiscal year		Fiscal year		Fiscal year	
Provider type	**2009**	**2013[a]**	**2009**	**2013[a]**	**2009**	**2013[a]**	**2009**	**2013[a]**
Psychiatrist	136	132	2	5	5	9	143	146
Psychologist	214	247	10	14	112	103	336	364
Mental health nurse[b]	38	65	57	53	2	28	97	146
Social worker	220	231	141	143	66	117	427	491
Other licensed provider	0	0	0	0	0	0	0	0
Total	608	675	210	215	185	257	1,003	1,147

Source: GAO analysis of Department of Defense (DOD) data. | GAO-15-184.

[a]Fiscal year 2013 values do not include civilian and contract providers assigned to military treatment facilities and subordinate clinics within the National Capital Region Medical Directorate because beginning in fiscal year 2011 this command began reporting as a separate entity.

[b]The mental health nurse category includes both mental health nurse practitioners and mental health registered nurses. In fiscal year 2009, DOD did not report separate employment information on these two types of mental health providers.

Table 7. Total Number of Navy Mental Health Providers, Fiscal Year 2009 Compared to Fiscal Year 2013

	Employment Category							
	Military		Civilian		Contract		Total	
	Fiscal year		Fiscal year		Fiscal year		Fiscal year	
Provider type	**2009**	**2013[a]**	**2009**	**2013[a]**	**2009**	**2013[a]**	**2009**	**2013[a]**
Psychiatrist	97	109	27	38	49	28	173	175
Psychologist	106	144	100	103	102	93	308	340

	Employment Category							
	Military		Civilian		Contract		Total	
	Fiscal year		Fiscal year		Fiscal year		Fiscal year	
Provider type	2009	2013[a]	2009	2013[a]	2009	2013[a]	2009	2013[a]
Mental health nurse[b]	69	103	13	16	118	77	200	196
Social worker	22	51	99	89	59	66	180	206
Other licensed provider	0	0	18	23	4	31	22	54
Total	294	407	257	269	332	295	883	971

Source: GAO analysis of Department of Defense (DOD) data. | GAO-15-184.

[a]Fiscal year 2013 values do not include civilian and contract providers assigned to military treatment facilities and subordinate clinics within the National Capital Region Medical Directorate because beginning in fiscal year 2011 this command began reporting as a separate entity.

[b]The mental health nurse category includes both mental health nurse practitioners and mental health registered nurses. In fiscal year 2009, DOD did not report separate employment information on these two types of mental health providers.

End Notes

[1] See GAO, Military Personnel: Enhanced Collaboration and Process Improvements Needed for Determining Military Treatment Facility Medical Personnel Requirements, GAO-10-696 (Washington, D.C.: July 29, 2010).

[2] Within DOD's health care system, servicemembers, dependents, and other beneficiaries can receive care both in DOD's own military treatment facilities (MTF) or through its TRICARE purchased care system of civilian providers. The TRICARE purchased care network is used to supplement the care provided by MTFs and MTFs may review all requests for specialty care, such as mental health care, to determine if they have the capability and capacity to provide the care.

[3] See Executive Order 13625, Improving Access to Mental Health Services for Veterans, Service Members, and Military Families (Aug. 31, 2012).

[4] In this report, we use the term mental health provider to describe a licensed or certified clinical provider—those that have met the minimum requirements needed to obtain and maintain a license or certification—including psychiatrists, psychologists, mental health nurse practitioners, mental health registered nurses, licensed social workers, and other licensed providers. We did not review other types of mental health personnel, such as administrative staff and technicians, who may not be licensed or certified but may be included in the population referred to by applicable laws. In this report we use the term mental health provider and mental health personnel interchangeably.

[5] See Congressional Budget Office, Approaches to Reducing Federal Spending on Military Health Care: Actual and Projected Costs for Military Health Care as a Share of DOD's Base Budget, 2000 to 2028, Pub. No. 4282 (January 2014).

[6] See Pub. L. No. 111-84, § 714, 123 Stat. 2190, 2381 (Oct. 28, 2009). The NDAA for Fiscal Year 2010 required DOD to increase the number of active duty mental health personnel. We discuss the status of these personnel increases in this report. The NDAA for Fiscal Year 2010 also required DOD to submit to Congress no later than one year after the enactment of the Act a report on the appropriate number of mental health personnel required to meet the mental health care needs of servicemembers, military retirees, and dependents. DOD issued this report to appropriate congressional committees in February 2011 and defined staffing levels for each service.

[7] NCR Medical Directorate manages DOD medical facilities within the national capital region. Military mental health providers working within NCR Medical Directorate facilities are accounted for in their military services' quarterly mental health staffing reports. However, the NCR Medical Directorate manages its own civilian and contract provider workforce and, as a result, reports its staffing levels separately from the military services for these two types of mental health providers.

[8] The Navy provides health care services for the Marine Corps.

[9] Section 723 of the NDAA for Fiscal Year 2006 directed the Secretary of Defense to establish a task force to examine Armed Forces mental health issues and produce a report containing an assessment of, and recommendations for, improving the efficacy of mental health services provided to servicemembers by DOD. The DOD Task Force on Mental Health was comprised of seven military and seven civilian professionals with mental health experience and issued its final report in June 2007. In August 2012, the President signed an executive order establishing an Interagency Task Force on Military and Veterans Mental Health, co-chaired by the Secretaries of Defense, Veterans Affairs, and Health and Human Services. This task force coordinates and reviews agency efforts to enhance veteran and military mental health and substance abuse services and develops recommendations on strategies to improve these services. See Executive Order 13625, Improving Access to Mental Health Services for Veterans, Service Members, and Military Families (August 31, 2012).

[10] See GAO, Defense Health Care: Department of Defense Needs a Strategic Approach to Contracting for Health Care Professionals, GAO-13-322 (Washington, D.C.: May 28, 2013). According to DOD, the MHS mission is to provide optimal health services in support of our nation's military mission—anytime, anywhere.

[11] In addition to operating its own health care facilities, DOD also provides health care to military servicemembers, dependents, and military retirees through its TRICARE purchased care network. TRICARE supplements the health care resources of DOD with networks of civilian health care providers.

[12] The Army and Navy each have a medical command, headed by a surgeon general, who manages each department's MTFs and other activities through a regional command structure. The Navy provides medical services for both Navy and Marine Corps installations. Unlike the Surgeons General for the Army and Navy, the Air Force Surgeon General exercises no command authority over Air Force MTFs; instead, Air Force MTF commanders report to local line commanders.

[13] Mental health provider totals in this report have been rounded to the nearest full-time equivalent. Information on mental health provider staffing levels contained in this report was obtained from quarterly mental health staffing reports submitted by the military services to DHA through the OASD HA human capital office.

[14] See Pub. L. No. 111-84, § 714, 123 Stat. 2190, 2381 (Oct. 28, 2009).

[15] This was in response to a September 2013 memorandum from the Assistant Secretary of Defense for Health Affairs that requested that the military services nominate their choice of

a mental health provider staffing model that would meet the following three criteria: (1) demonstrate adaptability to the Army, the Air Force, and the Navy; (2) demonstrate clinical validity to be used for the budget request to predict staffing; and (3) be ready for use for the fiscal year 2016 budget request. PHRAMS was the selected model for this process, which began in fiscal year 2014.

[16] DOD contracted with the CNA Corporation for the development and maintenance of PHRAMS.

[17] In addition to mental health providers, PHRAMS also includes estimates for the number of full-time equivalent primary care and other providers, including chaplains, needed by the MHS to administer mental health services. Primary care and other provider estimates are generated by PHRAMS because these providers deliver some mental health services to MHS beneficiaries.

[18] Some risk factors for dependents of servicemembers are populated based on their sponsoring servicemember's information.

[19] See L.M. Pikulin and D.M. Harris, The Psychological Health Risk-Adjusted Model for Staffing (PHRAMS): Update for Version 5.0, a special report prepared at the request of the Department of Defense, December 2013. PHRAMS is also used to estimate the number of TRICARE providers that will be needed to provide mental health services to beneficiaries enrolled in the TRICARE network.

[20] PHRAMS uses a number of mental health diagnoses in its calculations, including those in the following groups: (1) psychoses, (2) non-psychotic depressive disorders, (3) anxiety-related disorders, (4) neurotic disorders, (5) post-traumatic stress disorder, (6) adjustment reaction disorders (excluding post-traumatic stress disorder), (7) acute reaction to stress, (8) substance-induced mental disorders, (9) substance dependence, (10) non-dependent substance abuse, (11) psychotic disorders of childhood, (12) non-psychotic disorders of childhood, (13) schizophrenic disorder, (14) personality disorders, (15) disturbance of conduct not elsewhere classified, (16) other psychotic disorders, and (17) other non-psychotic disorders. PHRAMS also estimates the prevalence of a number of mental health related events, such as (1) personal or family history of mental or psychiatric diagnosis, (2) mental or behavioral problem influencing health status, (3) specific mental health circumstances, (4) mental health examination and observation with no reported diagnosis, (5) mental health condition in a mother complicating pregnancy, (6) post-deployment health assessments and post-deployment health reassessments, and (7) other cases where the diagnosing provider is a mental health provider.

[21] The model includes a small upward adjustment to each risk group's prevalence rate to account for untreated mental health conditions in the beneficiary population.

[22] To establish the encounter rates used in PHRAMS, the PHRAMS contractor created a composite encounter rate for each mental health condition included in the model based on five inputs: (1) recommendations from a Navy work group, (2) recommendations from an Air Force work group, (3) information gathered from reviews of clinical literature, (4) information gathered from reviews of clinical practice guidelines, and (5) other interviews. Encounter rates are also adjusted based on historical data.

[23] Military and civilian mental health providers have different amounts of hours they can devote to encounters each year. For example, the default value in PHRAMS version 5 for military mental health providers' clinical encounter time was set at 1,190 hours per year, while the default value for civilian mental health providers' clinical encounter time was set at 1,399. This difference accounts for the hours military mental health providers spend each year

performing military-specific duties not related to beneficiary care and differences in assumed productivity for military and civilian mental health care providers.

[24] While the NCR Medical Directorate was required to use PHRAMS for its fiscal year 2016 budget request, we focused our analysis in this section on only the military services.

[25] See GAO, Standards for Internal Control in the Federal Government, GAO/AIMD-00-21.3.1 (Washington, D.C.: November 1999).

[26] The Army legacy staffing model calculates mental health provider staffing needs for each Army MTF by determining the number of relative value units for each MTF and projects the number of providers that are necessary to produce the desired level of productivity for the following year. Relative value units measure the amount of time and effort it takes to treat a beneficiary.

[27] An Air Force official told us that Air Force mental health consultants are senior clinicians from a variety of specialties assigned as consultants to the Air Force Surgeon General to assist in staffing and other necessary operations.

[28] GAO/AIMD-00-21.3.1.

[29] DOD refers to staffing needs as requirements.

[30] See GAO/AIMD-00-21.3.1.

End Notes for Appendix I

[1] Mental health providers working within the MHS fall within three employment categories: (1) military providers, who can be either active duty or reserve servicemembers; (2) civilian providers; or (3) contract providers.

End Notes for Appendix II

[1] The Health Resources and Services Administration is an agency of the Department of Health and Human Services and is the primary federal agency charged with improving access to health care by strengthening the health care workforce, building healthy communities, and achieving health equity. The Health Resources and Services Administration designates certain areas of the nation as Health Professional Shortage Areas.

[2] The NDAA for Fiscal Year 2010 also included a number of other recruitment and retention mechanisms not highlighted in this report. These additional mechanisms included the expansion of DOD's capacity to train masters-level clinical psychologists and social workers with expertise in deployment-related mental health disorders, detailing commissioned officers to accredited schools of psychology for training leading to a doctoral degree in clinical psychology or social work, and reassigning military mental health providers from administrative to clinical positions.

[3] Qualifying HPSP students receive (1) full tuition for any accredited medical, psychiatric nurse practitioner, or psychology program; (2) a monthly stipend during the period of academic instruction; (3) officer's pay during academic breaks while training in DOD facilities; and (4) credit for time spent in educational training and placement in the appropriate rank as though this time was spent in active duty military service. Scholarship recipients incur a 1-year active duty military service obligation for each year they receive HPSP scholarship

payments, and minimum service obligations differ by health care field. Additional active duty service obligations may be incurred for residency and fellowship training.

[4] Generally, USUHS students do not pay tuition and receive full salary and benefits for a junior officer (second lieutenant or ensign) in exchange for a 7-year active duty military service commitment.

[5] Accession bonuses may be offered to certain new military servicemembers, including mental health providers. Retention bonuses, referred to in applicable laws and regulations as allowances, may be offered to existing military servicemembers and to current civilians, including mental health providers, if DOD determines that they have high or unique qualifications or DOD has a special need for the providers' services that makes it essential to retain them and the providers would be likely to leave federal service if a retention incentive was not offered. Relocation bonuses may be offered to current civilians, including mental health providers, who must relocate to accept positions in a different geographic area if the agency determines that their positions are likely to be difficult to fill in the absence of incentives.

[6] An Army official told us that the Army has begun discussions with the Air Force to train a small number of Air Force social work military providers through this program as well.

[7] The Health Resources and Services Administration designates certain areas of the nation as Health Professional Shortage Areas. Health Professional Shortage Areas may be urban or rural areas, population groups, or medical or other public facilities. In order for an area to be designated as a mental health Health Professional Shortage Area, there must be a psychiatrist to population ratio of at least 1: 30,000. In other words, when there are 30,000 or more people per psychiatrist, an area is eligible to be designated as a mental health Health Professional Shortage Area.

In: Staffing Issues in Military Health Care
Editor: Douglas Parker
ISBN: 978-1-63482-993-9

Chapter 2

VA HEALTH CARE: ACTIONS NEEDED TO ENSURE ADEQUATE AND QUALIFIED NURSE STAFFING*

United States Government Accountability Office

ABBREVIATIONS

FY	fiscal year
LPN	licensed practical nurse
NA	nursing assistant
NDNQI	National Database of Nursing Quality Indicators
NHPPD	nursing hours per patient day
OIG	Office of Inspector General
ONS	Office of Nursing Services
RN	registered nurse
VA	Department of Veterans Affairs
VAMC	VA medical center
VHA	Veterans Health Administration
VISN	Veterans Integrated Service Network

* This is an edited, reformatted and augmented version of The United States Government Accountability Office publication, GAO-15-61, dated October 2014.

WHY GAO DID THIS STUDY

GAO and others have raised prior concerns about the adequacy and qualifications of VHA's nurse staffing. In part to address these concerns, VHA issued a directive in 2010 requiring all VAMCs to implement a standardized methodology for determining an adequate and qualified nurse workforce, which includes developing and executing nurse staffing plans. It also requires VAMCs to use the methodology on an ongoing basis to evaluate staffing plans.

GAO was asked to provide information on nurse staffing at VAMCs. This report reviews the extent to which

1. VAMCs have implemented VHA's nurse staffing methodology, and
2. VHA oversees VAMCs' implementation and ongoing administration of the methodology. GAO reviewed documents and interviewed officials from VHA, seven VAMCs selected to ensure variation in factors such as geographic location, and regional offices for these VAMCs. GAO used federal internal control standards to evaluate VHA's oversight. GAO also interviewed representatives of veterans service organizations, nursing organizations, and unions.

WHAT GAO RECOMMENDS

GAO recommends VA: (1) assess VAMCs' ability to implement the methodology, (2) monitor VAMCs' ongoing compliance with the methodology, (3) complete timely evaluations, (4) improve the timeliness of communication with VAMCs, and (5) define areas of responsibility and reporting within VA's management structure. VA concurred with the recommendations.

WHAT GAO FOUND

The seven Department of Veterans Affairs medical centers (VAMC) in GAO's review implemented the Veterans Health Administration's (VHA) nurse staffing methodology, experienced problems developing and executing the related nurse staffing plans, and some reported improvements in nurse staffing. Specifically, GAO found that each of the seven VAMCs had developed a facility-wide staffing plan—which outlines initiatives needed to ensure appropriate unit-level nurse staffing and skill mix—and taken steps to execute it. However, VAMCs experienced problems—such as lack of data resources and difficulties with training—in both the development and execution of their staffing plans. Some VAMC staff reported improvements in the adequacy and qualifications of their units' nursing staff when nurse staffing plan initiatives were executed. For example, at two VAMCs where the number of nurses was increased or where support services for nurses were put in place, such as a designated group of staff to assist in transporting patients to and from appointments off the unit, unit staff said the adequacy of the nursing staff had improved. However, some VAMC unit staff reported that unit nurse staffing continued to be inadequate and that nurse unit assignments and job duties were not always appropriate for their qualifications.

VHA's oversight is limited for ensuring its nurse staffing methodology is implemented and administered appropriately. GAO found the following internal controls were limited in VHA's oversight process:

- *Environmental assessment.* VHA did not comprehensively assess each VAMC to ensure preparedness for implementing the methodology, including having the necessary technical support and resources, prior to the issuance of the directive requiring each VAMC to implement the methodology.
- *Monitoring compliance.* VHA does not have a plan for monitoring VAMCs to ensure compliance with the implementation and ongoing administration of the methodology.
- *Evaluation.* VHA has conducted limited evaluations of the methodology, and at least one of these evaluations has been significantly delayed.
- *Timeliness of communication.* VHA's protracted timeline for communicating methodology-related information may have hindered the ability of VAMCs to appropriately develop their staffing plans and to execute the initiatives contained in those plans.
- *Organizational accountability.* VHA did not define areas of responsibility or establish the appropriate line of reporting within VA's management structure for oversight of the implementation and ongoing administration of the methodology.

Without these internal controls in place, VHA cannot ensure its methodology meets department goals, such as establishing a standardized methodology for determining an adequate and qualified nurse workforce at VAMCs, and ultimately, having nurse staffing that is adequate to meet veterans' growing and increasingly complex health care needs.

* * *

October 16, 2014

The Honorable Mike Coffman
Chairman
Subcommittee on Oversight & Investigations
Committee on Veterans' Affairs
House of Representatives

Dear Mr. Chairman:

The Department of Veterans Affairs' (VA) Veterans Health Administration (VHA) provides medical care to millions of veterans each year. Nurses play an essential role in the medical care that veterans receive, and it is critical that VHA has an adequate and qualified nursing staff to meet veterans' needs. Studies have shown that better care is provided when facilities have both an adequate number of nurses, and nurses that are appropriately qualified for the jobs to which they are assigned.[1] According to VHA, it employs more than 80,000 nurses, making it the largest employer of nurses in the country. The number of veterans receiving care at VA medical centers (VAMC) increased from 5.2 million in fiscal year (FY) 2009 to 5.8 million in FY 2013, and VHA estimates that it will serve close to 8.8 million veterans by 2020. Furthermore, more intensive nursing care is being required by a growing number of veterans returning from military operations in Afghanistan and Iraq, and by aging veterans from prior eras of service.

For more than 10 years, concerns have been raised that VHA might not have an adequate and qualified nursing staff to care for the increasing number of veterans requiring more complex care. In 2002, Congress passed legislation requiring VA to develop a nationwide policy on staffing levels for the operation of VAMCs.[2]

Specifically, the law required VA to establish a nationwide policy on the staffing of VAMCs to ensure they have adequate staff, taking into account staffing levels and the mixture of staff skills required for providing care to veterans. The need for a new nurse staffing policy was highlighted in 2004 when VA's Office of Inspector General (OIG) issued a report raising concerns about the adequacy of nurse staffing levels in VAMCs' inpatient units.[3] By 2008, however, no national policy on nurse staffing had been implemented. In October 2008, we issued a report raising concerns about the adequacy of nurse staffing, specifically for registered nurses (RN) in inpatient units, and the need to expeditiously proceed with developing and implementing a new nurse staffing system, among other issues.[4] We recommended that VHA develop a detailed plan for implementing a new nurse staffing system and ensure it provided accurate nurse staffing estimates. In part to address these concerns, in 2010, VHA issued a directive requiring each VAMC to implement a nationally standardized methodology for determining an adequate and qualified nurse workforce, which includes the development and execution of nurse staffing plans. The staffing plans outline initiatives needed to ensure appropriate nurse staffing levels and skill mix in units to support high-quality patient care in the most effective manner possible. The directive also requires VAMCs to use the methodology on an ongoing basis to evaluate staffing plans at least annually.

You expressed interest in obtaining information on nurse staffing at VAMCs. In this report, we review the extent to which (1) VAMCs have implemented VHA's nurse staffing methodology, and (2) VHA oversees VAMCs' implementation and ongoing administration of its nurse staffing methodology.

To determine the extent to which VAMCs have implemented VHA's nurse staffing methodology, we reviewed documents and interviewed officials from VHA. Specifically, we reviewed information and interviewed officials from VHA's Office of Nursing Services (ONS)—the VHA office responsible for providing national policies, guidelines, and oversight for all VAMC nursing personnel—on the extent to which VAMCs have implemented the methodology in inpatient units (Phase I); VAMCs have piloted the methodology in operating room, emergency department, and spinal cord injury units (Phase II); and VHA has developed plans for an automatic staffing system (Phase III). We interviewed officials and nursing staff from seven VAMCs located in: (1) Battle Creek, Michigan; (2) Bronx, New York; (3) Columbia, South Carolina; (4) Dallas, Texas, (5) Fort Harrison, Montana; (6) San Diego, California; and (7) Tampa, Florida about their experiences implementing VHA's nurse staffing methodology. These VAMCs were selected to ensure variation in factors such as geographic location, rural versus urban location, complexity,[5] RN turnover rate, and Magnet status.[6] We did not independently assess the extent to which the VAMCs' implementation of the staffing methodology contributed to an adequate and qualified workforce. Furthermore, the results of our review of the seven VAMCs are not generalizable across all VAMCs. We reviewed literature and interviewed researchers who have published in the area of nurse staffing, representatives of selected veterans service organizations,[7] and representatives of selected nursing organizations and unions[8] to gain their perspectives about the current environment for nurse staffing, nurse staffing methodologies in general, and VHA's nurse staffing methodology.

To determine the extent to which VHA oversees VAMCs' implementation and ongoing administration of its nurse staffing methodology, we reviewed documents and interviewed officials from VHA. Specifically, we reviewed VHA documents, such as national directives, policies, and evaluation plans, to determine the extent to which VHA has provided VAMCs guidance regarding the implementation and ongoing administration of the staffing methodology. We interviewed officials from ONS, the seven VAMCs in our review, and the regional Veterans Integrated Service Networks (VISN)[9] for these seven VAMCs regarding their oversight of VAMCs' implementation of the staffing methodology. We also interviewed ONS officials and VAMC officials and staff about the extent to which VAMCs' implementation of the staffing methodology contributes to an adequate and qualified nurse workforce. To determine whether VHA applied appropriate internal controls in its oversight of the nurse staffing methodology, we used relevant criteria from federal internal control standards. We also used relevant strategic planning and performance measures from the Government Performance and Results Act as enhanced by the Government Performance and Results Modernization Act of 2010, as incorporated in GAO's guidance on assessing performance.[10]

We conducted this performance audit from September 2013 to October 2014 in accordance with generally accepted government auditing standards. Those standards require that we plan and perform the audit to obtain sufficient, appropriate evidence to provide a reasonable basis for our findings and conclusions based on our audit objectives. We believe that the evidence obtained provides a reasonable basis for our findings and conclusions based on our audit objectives.

Background

Nurse staffing is a critical part of health care because of the effects it can have on patient outcomes and nurse job satisfaction. According to VHA, its staffing methodology aims to maximize nurses' productivity and efficiency, while providing safe patient care by ensuring appropriate nurse staffing levels and skill mix.

VHA Nurse Workforce

VHA's nurse workforce is primarily composed of RNs,[11] licensed practical nurses (LPN),[12] and nursing assistants (NA). These nurses provide care—ranging from primary care to complex specialty care—in inpatient, outpatient, and residential care settings at 151 VAMCs across the country.[13] In addition to the size of the nursing workforce, the nursing skill mix—i.e., the share of each type of nurse (RNs, LPNs, or NAs) of the total—is an important component of nurse staffing. Units vary in their nursing skill mix, depending on the needs of their patients. For example, intensive care units require higher intensity nursing, and may have a skill mix that is primarily composed of RNs compared to other types of nursing units that may provide less complex care. (See table 1 for a general description of the types of nursing staff position, responsibilities, and educational requirements.)

Although the number of nurses at VAMCs increased from FY 2009 to FY 2013, VHA ranked nurses as the second most challenging occupation to recruit and retain. Specifically, the total number of nurses at VAMCs increased 13 percent from 72,542 in FY 2009 to 81,940 in FY 2013, with similarly proportionate increases within each position type—RN, LPN, and NA. During the same time period, the annual nurse turnover rate at VAMCs—the percentage of nurses who left VHA through retirement, death, termination, or voluntary separation—increased from 6.6 percent to 8.0 percent. Although RNs had the lowest turnover rate among nurses, VHA noted particular difficulty recruiting and retaining for the position, particularly for RNs with advanced professional skills, knowledge, and experience, such as RNs that provide services in medical and surgical care units. [14] VHA projects that approximately 40,000 new nurses will be needed through FY 2018 to maintain current staffing levels and to meet the needs of veterans.

Table 1. Types of Nursing Staff Position, Responsibilities, and Educational Requirements

Position type	Responsibilities	Educational requirements
Registered nurse (RN)	Assesses and provides care to patients, administers medications; documents patients' medical conditions, including admissions and discharges; analyzes test results; establishes treatment plans; and operates medical equipment.	Highest educational requirements: Has completed a nursing education program, met state licensing requirements, and passed a nurse licensing examination to obtain an RN license.
Licensed practical nurse (LPN)[a]	Takes patient vital signs, provides basic care, and administers medications, but generally does not provide certain complex patient care services such as patient assessments or administration of intravenous medications.	Fewer educational requirements than RNs: Has a high school diploma or its equivalent and passeda licensing examination upon completion of a state-approved program available at technical schools and community colleges, typically lasting 1 year.
Nursing assistant	Attends to basic patient needs such as providing personal care to patients (e.g., assistance with bathing, dressing, and personal hygiene), carries out non-specialized duties (e.g., measure blood pressure), and supports other nursing staff.	Less extensive educational requirements than RNs andLPNs: Has registered as a nursing assistant with their state health department, and passed a written competency examination upon completion of a state-approved training program, generally lasting 3 to 12 weeks.

Source: VHA, nursing organizations, and literature. I GAO-15-61.

[a] LPNs and licensed vocational nurses have the same level of education and patient care responsibilities. In this table, when we refer to LPNs, we are referring to both LPNs and licensed vocational nurses.

VHA's Nurse Staffing Methodology

To help ensure adequate and qualified nurse staffing at VAMCs, in July 2010, VHA issued *VHA Directive 2010-034: Staffing Methodology for VHA Nursing Personnel*. ONS, the VHA office responsible for providing national policies and guidelines for all VHA nursing personnel, led the development of the nurse staffing methodology, which began in 2007. (See fig. 1.)

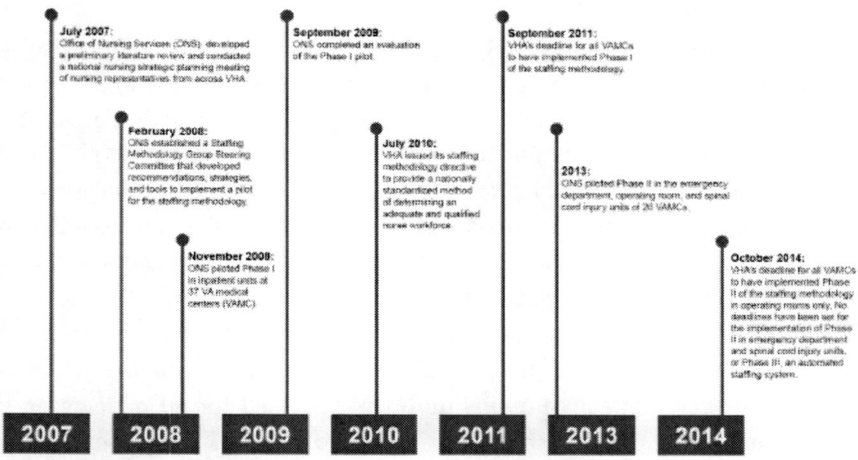

Source: VHA | GAO-15-61.

Figure 1. Timeline for Development and Implementation of the Veterans Health Administration's (VHA) Nurse Staffing Methodology.

To implement the methodology, each VAMC is required to (1) develop a VAMC-wide staffing plan for its nurse workforce, comprised of individual unit-level staffing plans, and (2) execute that plan. (See figure 2 for an outline of the process for implementing VHA's nurse staffing methodology.)

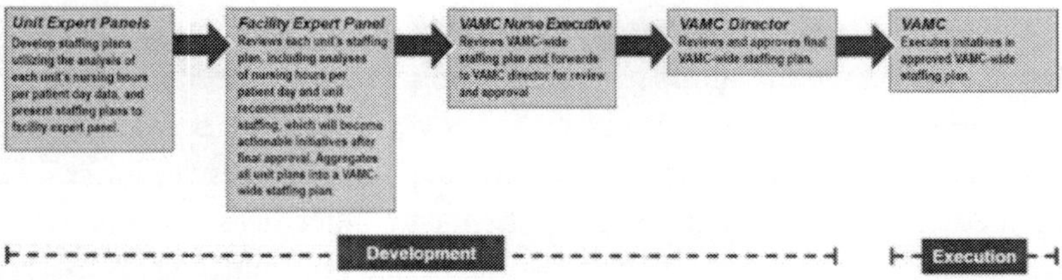

Source: VHA | GAO-15-61.

Figure 2. VA Medical Center (VAMC) Process for Implementing the Veterans Health Administration's (VHA) Nurse Staffing Methodology.

Each VAMC unit is to develop a staffing plan outlining recommendations on the appropriate nurse staffing levels and skill mix needed in that unit to support high-quality patient care in the most effective manner possible. Specifically, staffing plans are to be developed using expert panels and a data-driven analysis of nursing hours per patient day (NHPPD). VAMC nurse executives—members of senior management within each VAMC— are responsible for implementing the staffing methodology in their respective VAMCs.

- *Expert panels:* advisory groups—at the unit and facility level—of VAMC staff with in-depth knowledge of nurse staffing needs. The use of expert panels is intended to apply principles of shared governance, which allows nurses to have influence over the delivery of patient care and involves stakeholders from across the VAMC. VAMC nurse executives are responsible for ensuring that the unit-based expert panels represent all nursing types (RN, LPN, NA) and developing the VAMC's facility expert panel.
- *Data-driven analysis of NHPPD:* involves determining the number and skill mix of nurses needed for each unit by calculating the number of direct patient care nursing hours provided for all patients on that unit during a 24-hour period.[15] The use of NHPPD represents a move away from the more traditional nurse-to-patient ratios that assign a certain number of patients to each nurse. Some research suggests that NHPPD can better capture changes in nurses' workloads and case mix resulting from admissions and discharges, as well as patient acuity levels, which can impact the amount of time nurses spend with each patient.[16]

After developing the staffing plan, each unit-based expert panel presents its plan, which includes staffing recommendations, to the VAMC's facility expert panel. Those staffing recommendations may include, for example, initiatives to change the number and skill mix of nurses needed for each shift; change the number of nurses required for coverage during predicted absences, such as annual and sick leave; and develop support services for nurses, such as designated individuals to transport patients to other areas of the facility as needed. The facility expert panel—comprised of staff from across the VAMC—reviews each unit-based panel's staffing plan and aggregates all of the unit plans into one VAMC-wide staffing plan. The VAMC nurse executive reviews the VAMC-wide staffing plan and forwards it to the VAMC director for review and approval. Once approved, the VAMC then begins execution of the initiatives outlined in the VAMC-wide staffing plan. The directive requires each VAMC to conduct an ongoing staffing analysis to evaluate staffing plans annually, at a minimum, and for VAMC directors to incorporate projected staffing needs into their annual budget review.

The staffing methodology is being implemented in three phases.

- In Phase I, VAMCs were to implement the staffing methodology in all inpatient units no later than September 30, 2011.
- In Phase II, VAMCs are to implement the staffing methodology for all other units, including the operating room, emergency department, and spinal cord injury units.[17] ONS has completed the Phase II pilot for operating room units, and VAMCs are expected to implement the methodology in their operating room units by October 1, 2014. Deadlines for the implementation in other Phase II units have not been set.
- In Phase III, VAMCs are to use an automated system developed by VHA that (1) merges VHA staffing data used in the staffing methodology and other VHA data, such as human resource data, into one data system, and (2) incorporates the data into staffing-related reports, such as quality-of-care reports. A deadline for Phase III implementation has not been set.

In May 2014, the VA OIG found that VAMCs in its review varied in their implementation of the staffing methodology. Specifically, the VA OIG reported that 8 of the 28 VAMCs reviewed had not fully implemented all components of the staffing methodology by September 2013, 2 years past the implementation date required by the VHA directive.[18] As these findings were similar to those of its April 2013 report,[19] the VA OIG stated in its 2014 report, "We re-emphasize the need for all facilities to fully implement the methodology and accurately address patient needs with safe and adequate staffing."

Impact of Nurse Staffing on Patient Outcomes and Nurse Job Satisfaction

Adequate and qualified nurse staffing at VAMCs is required to provide effective and continuous patient care and to maintain a stable and engaged workplace. The importance of nurse staffing on patient outcomes and nurse job satisfaction has been emphasized by various entities, including The Joint Commission;[20] American Nurses Association;[21] Institute of Medicine;[22] and Agency for Healthcare Research and Quality.[23] Additionally, research has linked the adequacy and qualifications of nurse staffing to patient outcomes and nurse job satisfaction. For example, studies have shown:

- A link between the adequacy of nurse staffing and patient outcomes, particularly in inpatient units, such as intensive care and surgical units. For example, medication errors, pressure ulcers, hospital acquired infections, pneumonia, longer-than-expected stays, and higher mortality rates each have been associated with inadequate nurse staffing. 24
- A link between the qualifications of nursing staff and patient outcomes. For example, one study found that patients cared for in units utilizing more licensed and experienced nursing staff (RNs and LPNs) and fewer unlicensed aides (NAs) had shorter lengths of stay.[25] Other studies linked baccalaureate-prepared nurses to lower mortality rates.[26]
- A link between nurse staffing and job satisfaction. For example, some studies have linked low job satisfaction to heavy workloads and an inability to ensure patient safety.[27] Other studies found that improving nurse staffing and working conditions may simultaneously reduce nurses' burnout, risk of turnover, and the likelihood of medical errors, while increasing patients' satisfaction with their care.[28]

Non-VA health care organizations use various approaches to ensure effective nurse staffing. For example, some use fixed nurse-to-patient ratios while others use adjustable, unit-specific minimum staffing levels,[29] and there have been several efforts to address nurse staffing using these different approaches.[30] For example, California has enacted legislation requiring regulations that mandate specific nurse-to-patient ratios that limit the number of patients cared for by an individual nurse. Other states have passed legislation or adopted regulations addressing nurse staffing without mandating specific ratios or staffing levels. For example, some states require hospitals to have committees responsible for developing unit staffing plans or require public reporting of staffing.

VAMCs in Our Review Implemented VHA's Nurse Staffing Methodology, Experienced Problems Developing and Executing Staffing Plans, and Some Reported Improvements in Nurse Staffing

All seven VAMCs in our review developed staffing plans using VHA's nurse staffing methodology and have taken steps to execute them. However, VAMCs experienced problems in both the development and execution of their staffing plans. Improvements in nurse staffing were reported by some of the VAMCs which had taken steps to execute the staffing plans.

VAMCs in Our Review Have Implemented VHA's Nurse Staffing Methodology by Developing Staffing Plans and Taking Steps to Execute Them

The seven VAMCs in our review have implemented VHA's nurse staffing methodology; specifically, each of these VAMCs has developed a facility-wide staffing plan, comprised of unit-level staffing plans for inpatient units, and has taken steps to execute it.[31] Although each of the seven VAMCs in our review developed a staffing plan for FY 2013, only one had developed a plan per VHA's directive—that is, used both expert panels and analysis of NHPPD—by September 30, 2011, the deadline specified in the directive. (See table 2.) Across all 151 VAMCs, according to ONS officials, VAMCs' implementation of the nurse staffing methodology varied, with, for example, some VAMCs completing the development of their staffing plans during FY 2013, and some only beginning the development process.

In addition to developing staffing plans, all seven VAMCs in our review had taken steps to execute their respective staffing plans. For example, VAMCs had taken steps to execute initiatives to increase the number of unit nurses or change the skill mix of nurses to address patient care needs. (See table 3 for examples of VAMCs' staffing plan initiatives.) VAMC officials told us there are many factors that could affect the execution of staffing plan initiatives, such as available resources, the amount of time needed, and other strategic priorities.

Table 2. VA Medical Center (VAMC) Status for Development of VAMC-Wide Staffing Plan

		Status	
VAMC	*FY 2011*	*FY 2012*	*FY 2013*
A	●	●	●
B	o	●	●
C	o	●	●
D	o	o	●
E	o	o	●
F	o	●	●
G	o	●	●

Source: Seven VAMCs in our review. I GAO-15-61

● VAMC-wide staffing plan complete per Veterans Health Administration (VHA) directive.

o VAMC-wide staffing plan not complete per VHA directive.

Note: VHA Directive 2010-034 required each VAMC to develop a VAMC-wide staffing plan for use in its inpatient units by September 30, 2011. The process for developing the staffing plans included the use of expert panels—at the unit level and at the facility level—and a data-driven analysis of nursing hours per patient day.

Table 3. Examples of VA Medical Centers' (VAMC) Staffing Plan Initiatives

Initiative	Description
Number of nurses	Increase the total number of unit nurses—for example, registered nurses (RN), licensed practical nurses (LPN), or nursing assistants (NA)—to meet direct patient care needs.
Skill mix	Change skill mix of nurses to better meet patient needs—particularly having more RNs (rather than LPNs) to conduct timely patient assessments.
Contract nurse pool	Develop contracts to use temporary nursing staff from external employment organizations to meet short-term staffing needs.
Float pool	Develop designated group of nurses to float to units on an as-needed basis.
Sitter pool	Develop designated group of staff to provide one-on-one direct patient observation to allow nurses to bettercare for a broader group of patients.

Initiative	Description
Transport team	Develop designated group of staff to assist in transporting patients to and from appointments off the unit so that RNs are able to remain on the unit.
Staff reassignment	Reassign nursing staff from an overstaffed unit to an understaffed unit.
Patient census	Temporarily reduce patient census by closing beds because of inadequate staffing.

Source: Seven VAMCs in our review. I GAO-15-61.

VAMCs Experienced Problems Developing and Executing Staffing Plans, and Many of These Problems Persist

Officials and nursing staff from the seven VAMCs in our review told us they experienced problems developing and executing staffing plans. (See table 4 for examples of problems.) Some VAMCs were able to devise solutions; however in many cases, the problems have persisted.

Table 4. Examples of Problems VA Medical Centers (VAMC) Experienced Developing and Executing Staffing Plans

	Problems developing staffing plans					Problems executing staffing plans	
VAMC	Lack of necessary data resources	Difficulty completing and understanding training	Time required	Lack of communica-tion within VAMC	Difficulty integrating unit staff in expert panels	Hiring delays	Budget constraints
A		x	x			x	x
B	x	x	x	x	x	x	x
C	x		x	x	x	x	x
D	x	x	x	x		x	x
E	x	x	x			x	x
F	x	x	x	x	x	x	
G	x	x	x				

Source: Seven VAMCs in our review. I GAO-15-61.

Problems Developing Staffing Plans. Staff and officials from each of the seven VAMCs in our review reported facing problems developing staffing plans.

- *Lack of necessary data resources.* Staff and officials at six of the seven VAMCs in our review said they did not have the appropriate data resources to effectively calculate NHPPD as required by VHA's staffing methodology directive. Specifically, the directive instructs VAMC staff to calculate NHPPD using a wide range of data, such as number of admissions, transfers, and discharges; hours used for planning and treatment; and human resources data. We found that staff and officials needed to use multiple sources to collect the necessary data, in some cases manually, a process they said was time-consuming and potentially error-prone, and required data expertise they did not always have. For example, at one VAMC, the staffing methodology coordinator—a VAMC official who assists with the administrative tasks associated with the implementation process—told us she struggled with some data analysis techniques, such as creating a spreadsheet to help track staffing data, but the VAMC did not have the financial resources to hire additional data analysts to support the methodology. In contrast, officials from two VAMCs in our review told us staffing methodology coordinators were assigned in part based on their data analysis expertise.
- *Difficulty completing and understanding training.* Staff from six of the seven VAMCs in our review said the ONS training on the methodology was time consuming to complete, and difficult to understand. In 2011, ONS switched from instructor-led, group training to individual, computer-based PowerPoint training. Many unit staff reported that because the computer-based training took many hours to complete, it was difficult to find the time to complete it, while also carrying out their patient care responsibilities. They told us they often had to start and stop the training to attend to patients, which diminished its effectiveness. Further, the course's complex material was hard to absorb through an individual, computer-based course, with many staff suggesting their understanding would have been greatly improved with an instructor-led, group course where they could ask questions, ensure consistency of learning, and build camaraderie among unit expert panel members. To address the difficulties in completing and understanding the training, one VAMC

developed its own instructor-led, group training provided to all its units.

- *Time required.* Staff and officials at all seven of the VAMCs in our review reported that developing staffing plans required a lot of staff time due to the complexity of the process. In particular, they said gaining an understanding of the methodology, collecting the necessary data, convening the unit expert panels, and preparing presentations for the facility expert panel were time-intensive tasks that, in some circumstances, took time away from patient care. For example, members from one unit expert panel estimated they spent, in total, about 160 hours (4 weeks) developing the unit staffing plan during the first year the staffing methodology was implemented in their unit. Some VAMCs' staffing methodology coordinators developed specific processes designed to decrease the burden on nursing staff and improve efficiency. For example, they created templates for unit panel members to use in staffing plan development; such templates improved efficiency because unit panel members did not have to independently develop their presentation format. Further, facility expert panel members had to orient themselves to only one template, and were therefore able to more easily make facility-level comparisons and decisions.
- *Lack of communication within VAMC.* Unit expert panel members at four of the seven VAMCs in our review said there was a lack of communication between nurses and VAMC leadership regarding the status of the staffing plans, including plans for execution of the staffing plan initiatives. Staff at one of these VAMCs said they had not received any feedback on their FY 2012 or FY 2013 unit staffing plans; they added that developing the 2013 staffing plan without getting any feedback on the prior year's plan felt "frustrating." In contrast, at another VAMC, officials told us that all unit staff—not just staff involved in the unit panel—received regular updates on the nurse staffing process at their monthly unit staff meetings.
- *Difficulty integrating unit staff into expert panels.* Staff and officials at three VAMCs described challenges in integrating unit staff into expert panels. Some unit panel members told us that although they were considered members of their respective unit panels, they were not significantly involved in the development of their units' staffing plans. For example, a unit panel member said the VAMC's staffing methodology coordinator calculated the unit's NHPPD, developed the

corresponding unit staffing plan, and presented the unit staffing plan to the respective facility expert panel almost entirely without her unit's input. As a result, there was limited involvement of the unit panel members in the expert panel and, consequently, limited shared governance. Officials at these VAMCs said that from their perspectives, there was interest in the methodology among unit panel members, but sometimes it was difficult for these staff to attend relevant meetings because of patient needs. In contrast, unit panel members at other VAMCs in our review described how they were fully integrated into the unit panels. They described in detail the data analyses they prepared, the meetings they participated in, and their experiences presenting their unit staffing plans to the facility expert panel. Members from one unit panel told us it was helpful to be able to use data to validate the unit's staffing and share this data with the facility expert panel—VAMC staff "beyond the typical chain of command." Officials at this VAMC noted that unit panel members felt "empowered" to present their work to the facility expert panels.

Problems Executing Staffing Plans. Staff and officials from six of the seven VAMCs in our review noted problems executing staffing plans once approved by the VAMC director.

- *Hiring delays*. Staff and officials from six of the seven VAMCs in our review said they often faced hiring delays that impacted their ability to execute staffing plan initiatives. Some VAMC staff noted it could take more than 6 months to fill unit vacancies. Although staff from one VAMC said hiring was slowed by the dearth of qualified nurses in their community, staff from other VAMCs in our review said the supply of nurses was not the problem, but rather the problem was the VHA hiring process, which took months to complete for each candidate. Additionally, VAMC staff noted that new hires also needed to complete necessary internal trainings before joining a unit full time, which added to the delays, and that some new hires were hurried through this training process because their units were so desperate to have them on staff.
- *Budget constraints*. Staff and officials from five of the seven VAMCs in our review said their VAMCs were not able to fully execute their staffing plans due to budget constraints. For example, at one VAMC, one of the approved staffing plan initiatives was the hiring of a large

number of nurses for its units, in part, to address the VAMC's inability to increase their nursing staff over a period of years. The official told us that, due to budget constraints, the VAMC was going to phase in this hiring initiative over the next few years.

Improvements in Nurse Staffing Were Reported When VAMCs Executed Staffing Plan Initiatives

Some VAMC staff reported improvements in the adequacy and qualifications of their units' nursing staff when nurse staffing plan initiatives were executed. For example, at two VAMCs at which the number of nurses was increased or support services for nurses, such as patient transporters or sitters, were put in place,[32] unit staff said the adequacy of the nursing staff had improved. Furthermore, improvements in the qualifications of unit nursing staff were noted by staff in VAMC units where, for example, skill-mix changes were made or the amount of floating of nurses from their home unit to an unfamiliar unit was decreased. Both VAMC officials and unit staff noted improvements in staffing when nurses' qualifications were more appropriately matched to the right level of work (for example, having RNs rather than LPNs available to provide more complex patient care) and to the right units (for example, the units for which they were hired and trained).

Some VAMC staff said they also had seen improvements in patient outcomes and nurse job satisfaction. For example, nursing staff at one VAMC said that after creating sitter positions—as indicated by their VAMC's staffing plan—they saw a decrease in patient falls. The staff said sitters were able to monitor patients more closely, and as a result, patients were less likely to fall during walks to the bathroom, for example. Similarly, nursing staff in a mental health unit at another VAMC said that by having more staff they had decreased their restraint use because there were more staff available to meet veterans' needs. Additionally, nursing staff we interviewed at one VAMC that had made staffing changes based on staffing plans said they were better able to provide the type of nursing care "veterans deserve," and this made them feel more positive about their work. Some nurses at this VAMC also said the shared governance aspect of the methodology was empowering, which, combined with their enhanced understanding of staffing at their VAMC, helped improve their overall job satisfaction.

However, some VAMC unit staff reported that unit nurse staffing continued to be inadequate and that nurse unit assignments and job duties were not always appropriate for their qualifications. For six of the VAMCs in our review, staff from at least one unit interviewed said their unit staffing levels were inadequate. Staff said ensuring adequate staffing was particularly challenging when there were unplanned staff absences and they had to "scramble" to provide coverage. Some unit staff noted that this situation often resulted in units forcing nurses to work overtime or nurses floating to other units where they did not always have the qualifications to provide care. At some VAMCs, staff said there were increased staff injuries due to inadequate staffing. Furthermore, staff at one VAMC reported that where there had not been any changes made based on the unit staffing plans, their units continued to be understaffed to the detriment of both patient care and their job satisfaction.

VHA's Oversight to Ensure Its Nurse Staffing Methodology Is Implemented, Administered Appropriately, and Contributes to an Adequate and Qualified Nurse Workforce Is Limited

Our review of VHA's oversight of its nurse staffing methodology found that some internal controls—those related to environmental assessment, a plan for monitoring compliance, evaluation, timeliness of communication, and organizational accountability—are limited. The implementation of internal controls is necessary for ensuring initiatives achieve intended outcomes and for minimizing operational problems. Without these internal controls in place, VHA cannot ensure that its methodology meets department goals, such as establishing a standardized methodology for determining adequate and qualified nurse staffing at all VAMCs, and ultimately, having nurse staffing that is adequate to meet veterans' health care needs.

Environmental Assessment. VHA did not comprehensively assess each VAMC to ensure preparedness for implementing its methodology, including having the necessary technical support and resources, prior to the issuance of the methodology directive in 2010. Furthermore, as of August 2014, VHA did not have a plan for assessing whether VAMCs have the necessary resources to execute their approved nurse staffing plans. Under federal internal control standards, successful organizations monitor their internal and external environments continuously and systematically, and by building environmental assessments into the strategic planning process, are able to stay focused on long-term goals even as they make changes to achieve them.

VHA did not assess VAMCs' technical resources to determine if all VAMCs would be able to successfully implement the methodology. For example, the directive recommended that VAMCs use comparative data from external sources, such as the National Database of Nursing Quality Indicators (NDNQI) when analyzing unit-level staffing data. According to some VAMC officials, due to the costs and complexity of contracting,[33] not all VAMCs had access to this data source.[34] Each VAMC was responsible for establishing its own contract to purchase access to NDNQI data, which some VAMC officials said was expensive and time-consuming to set up, noting that it would have been helpful to have assistance in coordinating the contracting process. Officials from ONS reported that they are discussing the possibility of having a VHA-wide contract so that all VAMCs would have access to NDNQI data. In addition to access to comparative data, according to the directive, VAMCs need appropriate data system capabilities—in particular an automated staffing system for information such as patient admission, transfer and discharge data, and human resources data—to facilitate implementation of the data-driven methodology and calculation of NHPPD. However, not all VAMCs in our review had an automated staffing system in place even 3 years after the release of the directive. Officials at a VAMC without an automated staffing system told us staff were collecting and inputting data, in many cases manually, into a spreadsheet to calculate NHPPD, and that this process was extremely time-consuming and potentially error-prone. ONS officials said they knew VAMCs needed automated staffing systems when the directive was published in 2010. However, they thought Phase III—a national automated staffing system—would be forthcoming, and did not fully review whether VAMCs had alternative data capabilities to assist them in the interim.

When we asked how they assessed the readiness of VAMCs for implementation of the methodology, ONS officials told us that they did not do this as well as they should have for Phase I implementation in inpatient units, despite its 2009 Phase I pilot evaluation to better understand the potential capabilities and weaknesses of VAMCs. According to ONS, it still has not conducted such an assessment of all VAMCs even though it has moved forward with planning the national rollout of Phase II in operating room, emergency department, and spinal cord injury units. ONS, however, has assessed some of the available resources of the sites that have participated in the pilots for Phase II in spinal cord injury units. For example, ONS officials told us that they asked these participating sites questions about their access to data and nurse turnover within the pilot units to determine their ability to fully and successfully participate in the pilot. According to ONS officials, all sites reported that they were able to fully participate in the pilot. By not comprehensively assessing the VAMCs' technical support and resources to determine if they were prepared to implement the methodology, VHA had no assurance that the VAMCs would be successful.

Plan for Monitoring Compliance. ONS did not develop a plan for monitoring VAMCs to ensure they were in compliance with the implementation and ongoing administration of Phase I of the methodology. Under federal internal control standards, plans should be designed to ensure that ongoing monitoring occurs in the course of normal program operations, and managers should identify performance gaps in compliance with program policies and procedures.

ONS reported implementing two mechanisms for obtaining information from VAMCs—a 2013 questionnaire sent to all VAMCs and monthly methodology conference calls with VAMCs—but neither was an adequate mechanism for comprehensively assessing the compliance of each VAMC. The questionnaire, sent nearly 2 years after the deadline for implementation of Phase I of the methodology, asked VAMCs to report their status of staffing plan development, but because of lack of clarity in the questions asked, inconsistency in medical center responses, and lack of validation of the self-reported responses, it was not reliable for determining the extent to which VAMCs had developed staffing plans. ONS officials reported that they have no plans to survey VAMCs again on their status of developing staffing plans. Furthermore, the monthly methodology conference calls that started when the directive was published in 2010 did not provide an adequate mechanism for monitoring compliance because they too relied on VAMCs to self-report problems. A VAMC official told us that participants were reluctant to raise problems, such as not developing staffing plans on time, during these monthly calls.

In addition, the directive requires VAMCs to evaluate their staffing plans for Phase I annually, or more frequently if needed, but ONS officials told us that they did not have a systematic plan for monitoring compliance with this evaluation beyond the 2013 questionnaire and the monthly methodology conference calls. Moving forward, ONS officials said they plan to review whether all VAMCs implemented both the unit and facility expert panels, but, as of August 2014, had no detailed plan or timeline for conducting this review or for monitoring VAMCs' ongoing evaluation of their staffing plans. The lack of a plan for monitoring VAMCs' compliance with the implementation and ongoing administration of the methodology hinders VHA from being able to ensure that all VAMCs are staffing their nurses using the same, standardized methodology.

Evaluation. There have been limited evaluations of the methodology, and one of these evaluations has been significantly delayed. Under federal internal control standards, measuring performance allows organizations to track the progress they are making towards program goals and objectives, and provides managers important information on which to make management decisions and resolve any problems or program weaknesses.

- Evaluation of Phase I pilot (conducted in September 2009)—ONS identified VAMC challenges with implementing the methodology—such as difficulties accessing data, and staff nurses having an overall lack of knowledge of the methodology process. The evaluation contained recommendations, such as developing a training guidebook and providing guidelines on the role of the expert panels, to improve the methodology process. According to ONS, most of the recommendations from this 2009 evaluation have been addressed; however, we found that weaknesses identified in the 2009 evaluation still existed for all of the seven VAMCs included in our review.
- Evaluations of Phase I national implementation and training (began early 2014, preliminary results were expected August 2014). Similarly, ONS did not begin an evaluation of the national implementation of the methodology until January 2014, more than 2 years after VAMCs were required to have implemented it, and, as of August 2014, had still not been completed. According to ONS officials, the Phase I national evaluation was to review VAMCs' experiences during implementation, including a review of the training provided to VAMCs during that phase. The lengthy delay in the evaluation of Phase I was potentially problematic because the ongoing difficulties that VAMCs have experienced during implementation may have been avoided or resolved more quickly if the evaluation results had been available and corrective actions put into place. VAMC staff we interviewed told us they have been struggling with components of the methodology since the directive was issued. For example, some VAMC staff expressed difficulty completing and understanding the data analysis process for calculating NHPPD. An earlier evaluation of the methodology could have helped identify this problem, as well as potential solutions to address it. Furthermore, the

delay limited ONS's time to apply lessons learned from Phase I evaluations to the implementation of Phase II, portions of which are already nearly complete.

- Phase II pilot training evaluation (began in early 2014 with results expected November 2014)—ONS is conducting an evaluation of the training that was provided to the VAMCs involved in the Phase II pilots in operating room, emergency department, and spinal cord injury units to determine if the training provided to these units needs to be changed in preparation for the national rollout. ONS officials told us that they have completed the operating room pilot; the national rollout of the methodology in operating room units in all VAMCs began in February 2014 and is expected to be completed by October 1, 2014. ONS officials said that it has completed the pilot for the emergency department units, but has not completed the pilot for spinal cord injury units; ONS has not scheduled deadlines for their national implementation.

VHA's delays in completing evaluations of the methodology limit its ability to identify and resolve VAMC implementation and administration problems, and thus help to ensure successful rollouts of subsequent phases of the methodology.

Timeliness of Implementation and Communication. The long timeline for implementing the pilots and national rollouts of Phases I and II, as well as evaluating Phase I of the staffing methodology—more than 7 years— and for communicating methodology-related information to VAMCs may have hindered the ability of VAMCs to develop their staffing plans and to execute the initiatives contained in those plans. Under federal internal control standards, timeliness in the development of a program or implementation of a policy is needed to maintain relevance and value in managing operations and making decisions. When information regarding a policy or program is not provided in a timely manner, there can be a loss of stakeholder support, which can affect how stakeholders make decisions. For example, staff from some VAMCs involved in the Phase II pilot stated that they believed the data and reports generated from the methodology were only a paper exercise because they had not gotten any feedback from ONS on next steps. ONS officials told us they have communicated information on the Phase II pilot, such as the status of the pilot and feedback obtained from the training sessions, through their monthly conference calls with VAMCs; however, based on our interviews, this information did not reach many staff at the VAMCs in our review that participated in the Phase II pilot.

Furthermore, ONS officials have not adequately communicated to VAMCs the status of Phase III of the methodology—development of a national automated staffing system. According to the directive, a national automated staffing system was to be developed to support VAMCs in the implementation of the methodology. Because this automated staffing system has yet to be developed as per the directive, officials from two VAMCs told us they bought their own systems, which helped to effectively administer the methodology. ONS officials told us at the time the directive was published in 2010, Phase III implementation was an aspirational goal. ONS officials said they had expected VHA data system teams to begin the process of developing a national automated system; however, it was not made a department goal, and is not currently on the list of projects under consideration for funding. Having a variety of staffing systems, and thus inconsistent data variables across VAMCs, inhibits ONS's ability to adequately evaluate the effectiveness of the staffing methodology. If an automated staffing system is eventually developed under Phase III, VAMCs likely will have to dismantle the staffing systems they have created and restructure their data analysis processes, which likely will be time-consuming and costly. VHA's long timelines for the implementation and communication of methodology-related information put stakeholder support of the methodology at risk and increase the potential for duplication of efforts.

Organizational Accountability. VHA did not define areas of responsibility or establish the appropriate line of reporting within the framework of VA's management structure for the ongoing administration and oversight of the methodology. Under federal internal control standards, an agency's organizational structure should provide management with a framework for planning, directing, and controlling operations to achieve agency objectives; a good internal control environment requires that the agency clearly defines key areas of authority and responsibility. VHA does not require VAMCs to submit any information or reports on the implementation and ongoing administration of the methodology to ONS or the VISNs. Such information, if it were shared, may have been used to inform ONS of any systematic problems that necessitate changes to help ensure the continued viability of its methodology, as well as identify any best practices that have been implemented by VAMCs across the country. ONS officials told us that they did not require the VAMCs to submit any such documentation to ONS, because they made a conscious decision to not "micro-manage" the local process of nurse staffing.

Furthermore, VHA has not sufficiently utilized the VISN-level management structure in the implementation or ongoing administration of the methodology. While the methodology directive described a role for the VISNs, that role was limited to ensuring that resources are available to VAMCs as they try to staff their units; the directive did not mention a role in the implementation or ongoing administration of the actual methodology. As a result, VISNs have not been consistently aware of problems experienced by VAMCs in their region, and have not provided support or education. In our interviews with VISN officials representing each of the seven VAMCs in our review, we found that three of the VISNs were not substantively involved in the implementation and ongoing administration of the methodology. According to ONS, in many VISNs, discussions of staffing methodology implementation were minimal, and rather than VISN leadership, the nurse executives, in addition to their responsibilities within their individual VAMCs, had the responsibility of disseminating staffing methodology-related information to the VAMCs within the VISN.

Staff from three VISNs that were more substantially involved in the implementation of the methodology provided oversight for the nurse staffing methodology and acted as liaisons for VAMC nurse executives for network-level issues. One VISN official we interviewed was developing oversight mechanisms for VAMCs in the region, including a requirement for nurse executives to submit a quarterly staffing report. According to the official, having such a reporting requirement at the VISN level would give the right amount of emphasis to the process and provide support to nurse executives implementing the methodology in the VAMCs. The quarterly report could also help inform VISN officials about issues with the methodology. This official was developing these mechanisms independently of ONS, but they could be considered potential best practices to be shared across all VISNs.

ONS officials told us they thought ideas or problems across VAMCs related to the methodology would be shared through the VAMC nurse executives. They also hoped that VISN leadership would be interested in the methodology and, as a result, schedule VISN-level briefings to aid in its implementation. VHA, however, did not specify either of these roles in the directive or take steps to ensure that they were occurring. Moving forward, ONS officials said they are considering developing a VISN-level staff position that would specifically focus on educating VAMCs within the region about the methodology, and assisting them with implementing it. Without clearly defined roles and responsibilities within VA's organizational structure, VHA's ability to improve its oversight of the implementation and administration of the staffing methodology and provide VAMCs with additional resources to assist with problems is compromised.

CONCLUSION

As the number of veterans requiring care in VAMCs and the complexity of services needed by many of these veterans increase, the need for an adequate and qualified nurse workforce is increasingly critical. Although VHA's nurse staffing methodology was intended to provide a nationally standardized methodology for determining and ensuring adequate and qualified nurse staffing at VAMCs, its ability to do so across all 151 VAMCs is not likely to be realized unless existing weaknesses are addressed. Although some improvements in nurse staffing were reported with the implementation of the staffing methodology, the seven VAMCs in our review experienced problems developing and executing the related staffing plans, including problems pertaining to data resources, training, and communication. Many of these problems persist as the seven VAMCs continue to administer the methodology.

We also found that VHA's oversight of the staffing methodology is limited and in many cases lacks sufficient internal controls, which could diminish VHA's ability to ensure an adequate and qualified nurse workforce. In particular, VHA has not adequately assessed the needs or preparedness of VAMCs to effectively implement the methodology, does not have a formal mechanism to ensure VAMCs' ongoing compliance with the methodology, has not clearly defined a role in oversight for VISNs, and does not regularly communicate with VAMCs or VISNs to cull and share best practices system-wide. Furthermore, delays in VHA's evaluations of early phases of the staffing methodology have made them too late to be useful in designing future phases or helping VAMCs with implementation. Because the implementation and administration of the nurse staffing methodology is ongoing, it is critical that VHA improve its oversight to help ensure an adequate and qualified nurse workforce across all VAMCs.

Recommendations for Executive Action

To help ensure adequate and qualified nurse staffing at VAMCs, we recommend that the Secretary of Veterans Affairs direct the Interim Under Secretary for Health to enhance VHA's internal controls through the following five actions:

1. Provide support to all VAMCs to meet the objectives of the VHA directive, including:
   a) training that more clearly aligns with the needs of VAMC staff and
   b) a systematic process for collecting and disseminating staffing methodology best practices;
2. Conduct an environmental assessment of all VAMCs, including an assessment of their data analysis needs, to determine their preparedness to implement the remaining phases of the methodology, and use that information to help guide and provide the necessary support for the implementation of the remaining phases and for the ongoing administration of the methodology;
3. Develop and implement a documented process to assess VAMCs' ongoing compliance with the staffing methodology, including assessing VAMCs' execution of staffing plans and more clearly defining the role and responsibilities of all organizational components, including VISNs, in the oversight and administration of the methodology;
4. Complete evaluations of Phase I and Phase II and make any necessary changes to policies and procedures before national implementation of Phase II in all VAMCs; and
5. Improve the timeliness and regularity of communication with VAMCs, including unit-level staff, regarding the status of the various phases of the methodology.

Agency Comments

We provided a draft of this report to VA for its review and comment. In its written comments, VA generally agreed with our conclusions and concurred with all five of the report's recommendations. To address the recommendations, VA indicated that VHA will take a number of actions, such as developing a written document specifying its process for assessing ongoing compliance with the staffing methodology and improving the timeliness and regularity of communication with VAMCs through face-to-face regional training sessions. VA indicated that target completion dates for implementing these recommendations range from September 2015 through September 2016. Regarding the recommendation that VA complete evaluations of Phase I and Phase II before national implementation of Phase II in all VAMCs, VA indicated that, by September 2016, it would complete its evaluations and determine what opportunities exist to modify policies and procedures, but did not explicitly state that the evaluations would be completed before national implementation. We continue to emphasize the importance of completing the evaluations before national implementation of Phase II in all VAMCs.

Sincerely yours,
Debra A. Draper
Director, Health Care

End Notes

[1] See, for example, R.L. Kane et al., Nurse Staffing and Quality of Patient Care, Pub. No. 07-E005, March 2007, Agency for Healthcare Research and Quality; and Kaiser Permanente Institute for Health Policy, Nurse Staffing and Care Delivery Models: A Review of the Evidence (Menlo Park, Calif.: March 2002).

[2] Pub. L. No. 107-135, Title I, § 124, 115 Stat. 2446, 2452 (Jan. 23, 2002)

[3] See Department of Veterans Affairs, Office of the Inspector General, Healthcare Inspection: Evaluation of Nurse Staffing in Veterans Health Administration Facilities, 03-00079-183 (Washington, D.C.: Aug. 13, 2004).

[4] See GAO, VA Health Care: Improved Staffing Methods and Greater Availability of Alternate and Flexible Work Schedules Could Enhance the Recruitment and Retention of Inpatient Nurses, GAO-09-17 (Washington, D.C.: Oct. 24, 2008).

[5] VA assigns each VAMC a complexity score derived from multiple variables to measure facility complexity arrayed along four categories, namely: patient population served, clinical services offered, education and research complexity, and administrative complexity.

[6] Magnet status is a designation of the Magnet Recognition Program®—a nationwide program developed by the American Nurses Credentialing Center, a subsidiary of the American Nurses Association, to recognize health care organizations for quality patient care, nursing excellence, and innovations in professional nursing practice. To attain Magnet status, hospitals must meet certain requirements, related to areas including staffing practices and quality monitoring.

[7] We spoke with officials from the Disabled American Veterans and Paralyzed Veterans of America who are knowledgeable about nurse staffing methodologies in VAMC inpatient units, such as spinal cord injury units.

[8] We interviewed officials from the American Nurses Association. We also contacted each of the nursing organizations that VHA officials told us work with VA nurses: American Federation of Government Employees, National Nurses United, National Association of Government Employees, National Federation of Federal Employees, and Nurses Organization of Veterans Affairs.

[9] Each of VA's 21 VISNs is responsible for managing and overseeing VAMCs within a defined geographic area.

[10] GAO, Managing For Results: GPRA Modernization Act Implementation Provides Important Opportunities to Address Government Challenges, GAO-11-617T (Washington, D.C.: May 10, 2011); Executive Guide: Effectively Implementing the Government Performance and Results Act, GAO/GGD-96-118 (Washington, D.C.: June 1996); Standards for Internal Control in the Federal Government, GAO/AIMD-00-21.3.1 (Washington, D.C.: November 1999); Internal Control Management and Evaluation Tool, GAO-01-1008G (Washington, D.C.: August 2001); VA Dialysis Pilot: Increased Attention to Planning, Implementation, and Performance Measurement Needed to Help Achieve Goals, GAO-12-584 (Washington, D.C.: May 23, 2012); Managing For Results: Executive Branch Should More Fully Implement the GPRA Modernization Act to Address Pressing Governance Challenges, GAO-13-518 (Washington, D.C.: June 26, 2013).

[11] According to VHA, the workforce data for RNs also include RNs with advanced degrees such as nurse practitioners.

[12] LPNs and licensed vocational nurses have the same level of education and patient care responsibilities. For the purposes of this report, when we refer to LPNs, we are referring to both LPNs and licensed vocational nurses.

[13] VHA also employs nurses to work outside VAMCs, such as those employed within its administrative offices. These nurses were not included in our review.

[14] See Department of Veterans Affairs, Veterans Health Administration, 2013 Workforce Succession Strategic Plan (Washington, D.C.: 2013).

[15] VHA's directive defines direct patient care as all patient- or resident-centered nursing activities performed by staff assigned to the unit. These activities include nursing assessments, admission and discharge activities, and patient teaching and communication.

[16] J. Spetz et al., "How Many Nurses Per Patient?" Health Services Research, vol. 43 (October 2008):1674-1692; Carayon, P. and A. Gurses, "Nursing Workload and Patient Safety in Intensive Care Units: A Human Factors Engineering Evaluation of the Literature," Intensive and Critical Care Nursing, vol. 21 (2005): 284-301; and American Association of Critical-Care Nurses, Standards for Establishing and Sustaining Healthy Work Environments (Aliso Viejo, Calif.: American Association of Critical-Care Nurses, 2005).

[17] According to ONS officials, the staffing methodology for these units were to be implemented separately from those included in Phase I because of the potential need to modify the methodology to align with the special services these units provide.

[18] See Department of Veterans Affairs, Office of the Inspector General, Combined Assessment Program Summary Report: Evaluation of Nurse Staffing in Veterans Health Administration Facilities April – September 2013, Report No. 14-01072-140 (Washington, D.C.: May 12, 2014).

[19] See Department of Veterans Affairs, Office of the Inspector General, Combined Assessment Program Summary Report: Evaluation of Nurse Staffing in Veterans Health Administration Facilities, Report No. 13-01744-187 (Washington, D.C.: April 30, 2013).

[20] Joint Commission on Accreditation of Healthcare Organizations, Health Care at the Crossroads: Strategies for Addressing the Evolving Nursing Crisis (Chicago, Ill.: Joint Commission on Accreditation of Healthcare Organizations, 2002).

[21] See American Nurses Association, Principles for Nurse Staffing, Second Edition (Silver Spring, Md.: American Nurses Association, 2012).

[22] Institute of Medicine, The Future of Nursing: Leading Change, Advancing Health (Washington, D.C.: The National Academies Press, 2011).

[23] See R.L. Kane et al., Nurse Staffing and Quality of Patient Care, Pub. No. 07-E005, March 2007, Agency for Healthcare Research and Quality; and "Hospital Nurse Staffing and Quality of Care," Agency for Healthcare Research and Quality, Research in Action, Issue 14, Pub. No. 04-0029 (Rockville, Md.: 2004).

[24] M.A. Blegen et al., "Nurse Staffing Effects on Patient Outcomes: Safety-Net and NonSafety-Net Hospitals," Medical Care, vol. 49, issue 2 (April 2011), 406–414; J. Needleman et al., "Nurse Staffing and Inpatient Hospital Mortality," New England Journal of Medicine, vol. 364, issue 11 (March 2011), 1037-1045; L.H. Aiken et al., "Implications of the California Nurse Staffing Mandate for Other States," Health Services Research, vol. 45, issue 4 (April 2010), 904–921; and P.W. Stone et al., "Nurse Working Conditions and Patient Safety Outcomes," Medical Care, vol. 45, issue 6 (June 2007), 571-578.

[25] A.P. Bartel et al., "Human Capital and Productivity in a Team Environment: Evidence from the Healthcare Sector," American Economic Journal: Applied Economics, vol. 6, issue 2 (2014), 231-259.

[26] A. Kutney-Lee, D.M. Sloane, and L.H. Aiken, "An Increase In The Number Of Nurses with Baccalaureate Degrees Is Linked To Lower Rates Of Postsurgery Mortality," Health Affairs, vol. 32, issue. 3 (March 2013), 579-586; L.H. Aiken et al., "Effects of Hospital Care Environment on Patient Mortality and Nurse Outcomes," Journal of Nursing Administration, vol. 38, issue 5 (May 2008), 223-229; and C.R. Friese et al., "Hospital Nurse Practice Environments and Outcomes for Surgical Oncology Patients," Health Services Research, vol. 43, issue 4 (August 2008), 1145-1163.

[27] J. Spetz, "Nurse Satisfaction and the Implementation of Minimum Nurse Staffing Regulations," Policy, Politics, & Nursing Practice, vol. 9 (Feb. 2008, first published on April 3, 2008), 15-21; and L.H. Aiken et al., "Hospital Nurse Staffing and Patient Mortality, Nurse Burnout, and Job Dissatisfaction," The Journal of the American Medical Association, vol. 288, issue 16 (October 2002), 1987-1993.

[28] A.W. Stimpfel, D.M. Sloane, and L.H. Aiken, "The Longer the Shifts for Hospital Nurses, the Higher the Levels of Burnout and Patient Dissatisfaction," Health Affairs, vol. 31, issue 11 (November 2012), 2501-2509; J.P. Cimiotti et al., "Nurse Staffing, Burnout, and Health Care-Associated Infection," American Journal of Infection Control, vol. 40 (August 2012) 486-490; and D.C. Vahey et al., "Nurse Burnout and Patient Satisfaction," Medical Care, vol. 42, issue 2 (Feb. 2004), 57-66.

[29] Fixed nurse-to-patient ratios assign a certain number of patients to each nurse (e.g., one nurse for every five patients) while adjustable, unit-specific, minimum staffing levels assign minimum ratios of nurses to patients for each unit and shift that reflects the needs of the patient population and matches the skills and experience of the staff.

[30] These are illustrative examples of different approaches; we did not conduct a comprehensive review of all state requirements.

[31] As previously described, VAMCs were required to implement the methodology in inpatient units (Phase I) no later than September 30, 2011. VAMCs were expected to implement the

methodology in their operating rooms by October 1, 2014; requirements for implementation of Phase II in other units and Phase III of the methodology have not been set.

[32] Transport teams are staff who assist in transporting patients to and from appointments off the unit. Sitters are staff who provide one-on-one direct patient observation.

[33] NDNQI was created as part of the American Nurses Association's Patient Safety and Quality Initiative to identify the linkages between staffing and patient outcomes. The database contains data on quality indicators and staff levels collected from approximately 2,000 hospitals that submit data on nursing-sensitive indicators, such as pressure ulcers and patient falls. According to the American Nurses Association, 98 percent of all Magnet facilities use some aspect of NDNQI data.

[34] According to the staffing methodology directive, a comparative analysis of NHPPD data from other resources is also recommended, such as from the Labor Management Institute and NDNQI. Labor Management Institute data compare direct, indirect, and total worked hours of care by hospital and unit type, and NDNQI data contain information on quality indicators and staff levels.

INDEX

J

L

M

N

O

P

Q

R

S

T

U

V

W